Growth, Somatic Maturation and Their Impact on Physical Health and Sports Performance

Growth, Somatic Maturation and Their Impact on Physical Health and Sports Performance

Editors

Francesco Campa
Gianpiero Greco

MDPI • Basel • Beijing • Wuhan • Barcelona • Belgrade • Manchester • Tokyo • Cluj • Tianjin

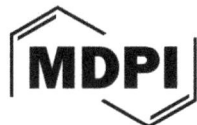

Editors
Francesco Campa
Department for Life Quality Studies
Università degli Studi di Bologna
Rimini
Italy

Gianpiero Greco
Department of Basic Medical Sciences, Neuroscience and Sense Organs
University of Study of Bari
Bari
Italy

Editorial Office
MDPI
St. Alban-Anlage 66
4052 Basel, Switzerland

This is a reprint of articles from the Special Issue published online in the open access journal *International Journal of Environmental Research and Public Health* (ISSN 1660-4601) (available at: www.mdpi.com/journal/ijerph/special_issues/GSMPPS).

For citation purposes, cite each article independently as indicated on the article page online and as indicated below:

LastName, A.A.; LastName, B.B.; LastName, C.C. Article Title. *Journal Name* **Year**, *Volume Number*, Page Range.

ISBN 978-3-0365-3087-1 (Hbk)
ISBN 978-3-0365-3086-4 (PDF)

© 2022 by the authors. Articles in this book are Open Access and distributed under the Creative Commons Attribution (CC BY) license, which allows users to download, copy and build upon published articles, as long as the author and publisher are properly credited, which ensures maximum dissemination and a wider impact of our publications.

The book as a whole is distributed by MDPI under the terms and conditions of the Creative Commons license CC BY-NC-ND.

Contents

About the Editors . . . . **vii**

Preface to "Growth, Somatic Maturation and Their Impact on Physical Health and Sports Performance" . . . . **ix**

Francesco Campa and Gianpiero Greco
Growth, Somatic Maturation, and Their Impact on Physical Health and Sports Performance: An Editorial
Reprinted from: *Int. J. Environ. Res. Public Health* **2022**, *19*, 1266, doi:10.3390/ijerph19031266 . . . **1**

Ana Filipa Silva, Sümer Alvurdu, Zeki Akyildiz, Georgian Badicu, Gianpiero Greco and Filipe Manuel Clemente
Variations of the Locomotor Profile, Sprinting, Change-of-Direction, and Jumping Performances in Youth Soccer Players: Interactions between Playing Positions and Age-Groups
Reprinted from: *Int. J. Environ. Res. Public Health* **2022**, *19*, 998, doi:10.3390/ijerph19020998 . . . **5**

Jelena Ivanović, Filip Kukić, Gianpiero Greco, Nenad Koropanovski, Saša Jakovljević and Milivoj Dopsaj
Specific Physical Ability Prediction in Youth Basketball Players According to Playing Position
Reprinted from: *Int. J. Environ. Res. Public Health* **2022**, *19*, 977, doi:10.3390/ijerph19020977 . . . **19**

Eileen Africa, Odelia Van Stryp and Martin Musálek
The Influence of Cultural Experiences on the Associations between Socio-Economic Status and Motor Performance as Well as Body Fat Percentage of Grade One Learners in Cape Town, South Africa
Reprinted from: *Int. J. Environ. Res. Public Health* **2021**, *19*, 121, doi:10.3390/ijerph19010121 . . . **31**

Jelena Slankamenac, Dusko Bjelica, Damjan Jaksic, Tatjana Trivic, Miodrag Drapsin and Sandra Vujkov et al.
Somatotype Profiles of Montenegrin Karatekas: An Observational Study
Reprinted from: *Int. J. Environ. Res. Public Health* **2021**, *18*, 12914, doi:10.3390/ijerph182412914 . **45**

Marina Saldanha da Silva Athayde, Rafael Lima Kons, David Hideyoshi Fukuda and Daniele Detanico
Body Size Measurements and Physical Performance of Youth Female Judo Athletes with Differing Menarcheal Status
Reprinted from: *Int. J. Environ. Res. Public Health* **2021**, *18*, 12829, doi:10.3390/ijerph182312829 . **55**

Alfonso Penichet-Tomas, Basilio Pueo, Sergio Selles-Perez and Jose M. Jimenez-Olmedo
Analysis of Anthropometric and Body Composition Profile in Male and Female Traditional Rowers
Reprinted from: *Int. J. Environ. Res. Public Health* **2021**, *18*, 7826, doi:10.3390/ijerph18157826 . . . **65**

Marcus Vinicius de Oliveira Cattem, Bruna Taranto Sinforoso, Francesco Campa and Josely Correa Koury
Bioimpedance Vector Patterns according to Age and Handgrip Strength in Adolescent Male and Female Athletes
Reprinted from: *Int. J. Environ. Res. Public Health* **2021**, *18*, 6069, doi:10.3390/ijerph18116069 . . . **77**

Sunghe Ha, Hee Seong Jeong, Sang-Kyoon Park and Sae Yong Lee
Can Neurocognitive Function Predict Lower Extremity Injuries in Male Collegiate Athletes?
Reprinted from: *Int. J. Environ. Res. Public Health* **2020**, *17*, 9061, doi:10.3390/ijerph17239061 . . . **89**

Carles Miguel Guillem, Andrés Felipe Loaiza-Betancur, Tamara Rial Rebullido, Avery D. Faigenbaum and Iván Chulvi-Medrano
The Effects of Resistance Training on Blood Pressure in Preadolescents and Adolescents: A Systematic Review and Meta-Analysis
Reprinted from: *Int. J. Environ. Res. Public Health* **2020**, *17*, 7900, doi:10.3390/ijerph17217900 . . . **103**

Hyun-Chul Jeong and Wi-Young So
Difficulties of Online Physical Education Classes in Middle and High School and an Efficient Operation Plan to Address Them
Reprinted from: *Int. J. Environ. Res. Public Health* **2020**, *17*, 7279, doi:10.3390/ijerph17197279 . . . **115**

João Pedro Nunes, Jeferson L. Jacinto, Alex S. Ribeiro, Jerry L. Mayhew, Masatoshi Nakamura and Danila M. G. Capel et al.
Placing Greater Torque at Shorter or Longer Muscle Lengths? Effects of Cable vs. Barbell Preacher Curl Training on Muscular Strength and Hypertrophy in Young Adults
Reprinted from: *Int. J. Environ. Res. Public Health* **2020**, *17*, 5859, doi:10.3390/ijerph17165859 . . . **127**

About the Editors

Francesco Campa

Francesco Campa, an adjunct professor at the Department of Life Quality Studies at the University of Bologna (Italy), received his PhD in pharmacology and toxicology, human development, and movement sciences from the University of Bologna. He has published one book on sports anthropometry, several book chapters, and over 60 peer-reviewed journal and conference papers (https://orcid.org/0000-0002-3028-7802), with an H-index of 15. His main interests are sports anthropometry, bioimpedance vector analysis, and body composition optimization applied to sports performance.

Gianpiero Greco

Gianpiero Greco has a PhD in neuroscience and translational medicine. His research fields focus on physical activity, physical education, exercise physiology, body composition, psychophysical health promotion, human performance, nutrition, special education, sport psychology, sport sociology, inclusive education, research methodology, and data analysis and involve the general population of all age groups, students, athletes, workers, and the tactical population.

Preface to "Growth, Somatic Maturation and Their Impact on Physical Health and Sports Performance"

Over time, complex interactions and a nonlinear progression among a wide range of variables contribute to improvements in the physical health and level of achievement in youth sports practitioners. Various elements, including technical skills, physical performance, environmental circumstances, and social conditioning, contribute to the development of these processes.

An influencing factor of growth and physical performance is somatic maturation. The pubertal period is a critical time for skill acquisition and improvements in performance for young people, in which suitable training strategies should be adopted to preserve their state of health while avoiding risks of injury. Athletes with similar chronological ages competing in the same category levels can, in fact, show differences in maturity and, therefore, in size, function, and body structure. Physical and psychological differences related to maturity and birthdate amongst athletes of the same selection year have been identified in a variety of sports and could be linked with the dropout of youth practitioners and a reduction in the talent pool.

Contemporary researchers have contributed to research on improving health and sports performance through the development of new measurement methods and training strategies in young athletes. The aim of this Special Issue of , entitled , Somatic Maturation, and Their Impact on Physical Health and Sports Performance, is to propose and evaluate new training strategies aimed at improving the health status and physical performance of young athletes while highlighting the relationship between somatic maturation, anthropometry features, education, and health-related factors via longitudinal and cross-sectional studies.

Francesco Campa, Gianpiero Greco
Editors

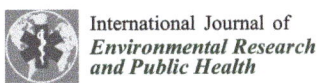

Editorial

Growth, Somatic Maturation, and Their Impact on Physical Health and Sports Performance: An Editorial

Francesco Campa [1],* and Gianpiero Greco [2]

1. Department of Biomedical and Neuromotor Sciences, University of Bologna, 40126 Bologna, Italy
2. Department of Basic Medical Sciences, Neuroscience and Sense Organs, University of Study of Bari, 70121 Bari, Italy; gianpierogreco.phd@yahoo.com
* Correspondence: Francesco.campa3@unibo.it

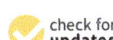

Citation: Campa, F.; Greco, G. Growth, Somatic Maturation, and Their Impact on Physical Health and Sports Performance: An Editorial. *Int. J. Environ. Res. Public Health* 2022, 19, 1266. https://doi.org/10.3390/ijerph19031266

Received: 17 January 2022
Accepted: 20 January 2022
Published: 24 January 2022

Publisher's Note: MDPI stays neutral with regard to jurisdictional claims in published maps and institutional affiliations.

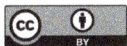

Copyright: © 2022 by the authors. Licensee MDPI, Basel, Switzerland. This article is an open access article distributed under the terms and conditions of the Creative Commons Attribution (CC BY) license (https://creativecommons.org/licenses/by/4.0/).

Over time, complex interactions and a nonlinear progression among a wide range of variables contribute to the improvement of physical health and of the elite level achievement in youth sport practitioners. Various elements, including technical skills, physical performance, environmental circumstances, and social conditioning, contribute to the development of these processes [1,2].

An influencing factor of growth and physical performance is somatic maturation [3,4]. The pubertal period is a critical time frame for skill acquisition and the development of performance in young people, in which suitable training strategies should be adopted to preserve the state of health while avoiding the risk of injury [5]. Athletes with similar chronological age competing in the same category levels can, in fact, show a difference in maturity status, and therefore in size, function, and body structure [6,7]. Physical and psychological differences related to maturity status and birthdate amongst athletes of the same selection year have been identified in a variety of sports and could be linked with the dropout of youth practitioners and a reduction in the talent pool [6].

Contemporary researchers have contributed to research on improving health and sports performance through the development of new measurement methods and training strategies in young athletes [8,9]. The aim of this Special Issue of *IJERPH* entitled Growth, Somatic Maturation, and Their Impact on Physical Health and Sports Performance [10] is to propose and evaluate new training strategies aimed at improving the health status and physical performance of young athletes while highlighting the relationship between somatic maturation, anthropometry features, education, and health-related factors via longitudinal and cross-sectional studies.

A total of 11 manuscripts are published here on different topics related to youth subjects and sports practice, as shown in Figure 1. Three papers are on physical performance aspects [11–13], five papers provide innovative findings in relation to anthropometry and body composition features [14–18], one paper examines the difficulties of running online physical education classes in the context of COVID-19 [19], and two are on the influence of training strategies on muscle strength and blood pressure [20,21].

Concerning physical and sports performance, Silva et al. [11] revealed that chronological age plays a determinant effect on vertical jump, linear sprint, and change of direction, revealing that older soccer players achieve better performance. On the contrary, playing position is not determined by age. Different player roles in youth basketball players were considered in the study of Ivanovic and co-workers [12]. The authors showed that (i) change of direction speed is the highest-ranked characteristic in basketball guards; (ii) jump performance is the highest-ranked feature in forwards; (iii) control of specific movements while dribbling the ball is the higher-ranked aspect in centers. Lastly, Ha et al. [13] demonstrated that neurocognitive function tests should not be used to predict lower extremity injuries in collegiate athletes.

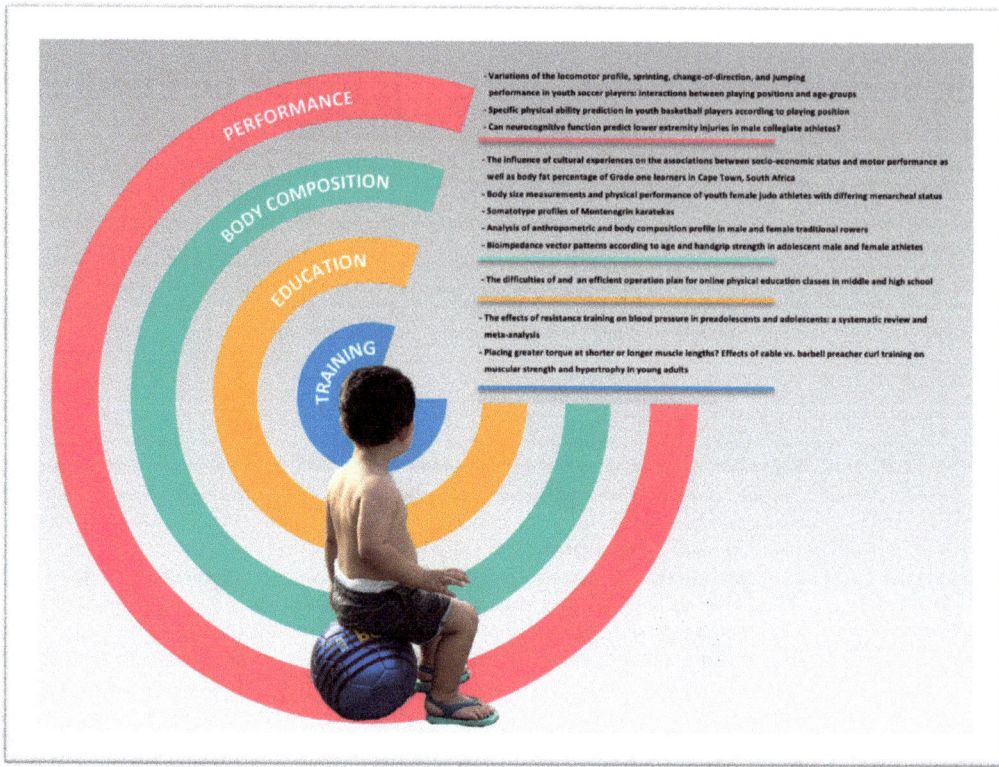

Figure 1. List of papers published in this Special Issue of IJERPH entitled Growth, Somatic Maturation, and Their Impact on Physical Health and Sports Performance [10].

Most of the papers published in this Special Issue focus on body composition, growth, and sports practice. In fact, body composition assessment is an important practice in sports management [22,23], given its numerous implications on the health and physical performance of youth subjects [24]. Obesity, child motor development, and physical fitness are influenced by socioeconomic status. In fact, Africa et al. [14] showed that in contrast to Western countries, children with lower socioeconomic status are leaner with a lower body fat and have better locomotor skills compared to their higher socioeconomic status peers in South Africa. Slankamenac et al. [16] provided specific somatotype profiles for Montenegrin karatekas, highlighting the peculiarities in body shape among different age and weight categories. Similarly, Penichet-Tomas et al. [17] published anthropometric references for male and female traditional rowers. The effect of age on body composition was also evaluated by Cattem and colleagues [18] in male and female athletes, who reported that subjects older than 13 years exhibited high fluid content and cell mass using qualitative and quantitative bioimpedance-based assessments. These data should be carefully considered in when developing training programs and talent selection procedures. In addition, Athayde et al. [15] reported that age at menarche and somatic growth are the primary indicators of physical performance in young female judo athletes.

Only one study examined the difficulties of running online physical education classes in the context of COVID-19 and used the findings to develop an efficient operation plan to address these difficulties [19]. The authors suggested that changes in strategic learning methods are needed to understand online physical education characteristics and thereby better communicate the value of physical education. They reported that it is necessary to cultivate teaching expertise through sharing online physical education classes, where collaboration among physical education teachers is central. In addition, the authors suggested that the evaluation processes should be less formal to encourage active student participation.

Two studies concerned resistance training practice and its effect on muscle strength and blood pressure in adolescents and young adults. Gullielm et al. [20] systematically reviewed and meta-analyzed the current evidence for the effects of resistance training on blood pressure in children and adolescents, concluding that this kind of exercise has no adverse effects on blood pressure and may positively affect it in youths. Lastly, Nunes et al. [21] suggested that biceps brachii muscle adaptations following a 10-week training program is almost identical regardless of whether peak torque emphasis was carried out in the final degrees or initial degrees of the range of motion in young adults.

In conclusion, as well as growth and development impacting children's sporting experience and physical characteristics, sports practice can also impact children's development and performance. This Special Issue reveals that the evolution of a healthy and successful athlete has a multifaceted nature and that several evaluation and training strategies are currently available to practitioners.

Author Contributions: Conceptualization, F.C. and G.G.; writing—original draft preparation, F.C.; writing—review and editing, G.G. All authors have read and agreed to the published version of the manuscript.

Funding: This research received no external funding.

Institutional Review Board Statement: Not applicable.

Informed Consent Statement: Not applicable.

Data Availability Statement: Not applicable.

Conflicts of Interest: The authors declare no conflict of interest.

References

1. Silva, A.M. Structural and functional body components in athletic health and performance phenotypes. *Eur. J. Clin. Nutr.* **2019**, *73*, 215–224. [CrossRef] [PubMed]
2. Campa, F.; Piras, A.; Raffi, M.; Toselli, S. Functional Movement Patterns and Body Composition of High-Level Volleyball, Soccer, and Rugby Players. *J. Sport Rehabil.* **2019**, 740–745. [CrossRef] [PubMed]
3. Campa, F.; Silva, A.M.; Iannuzzi, V.; Mascherini, G.; Benedetti, L.; Toselli, S. The Role of Somatic Maturation on Bioimpedance Patterns and Body Composition in Male Elite Youth Soccer Players. *Int. J. Environ. Res. Public Health* **2019**, *16*, 4711. [CrossRef] [PubMed]
4. Towlson, C.; Cobley, S.; Parkin, G.; Lovell, R. When does the influence of maturation on anthropometric and physical fitness characteristics increase and subside? *Scand. J. Med. Sci. Sports* **2018**, *28*, 1946–1955. [CrossRef]
5. Monasterio, X.; Gil, S.M.; Bidaurrazaga-Letona, I.; Lekue, J.A.; Santisteban, J.M.; Diaz-Beitia, G.; Lee, D.-J.; Zumeta-Olaskoaga, L.; Martin-Garetxana, I.; Bikandi, E.; et al. The burden of injuries according to maturity status and timing: A two-decade study with 110 growth curves in an elite football academy. *Eur. J. Sport Sci.* **2021**, 1–11. [CrossRef]
6. Toselli, S.; Campa, F.; Maietta Latessa, P.; Greco, G.; Loi, A.; Grigoletto, A.; Zaccagni, L. Differences in Maturity and Anthropometric and Morphological Characteristics among Young Male Basketball and Soccer Players and Non-Players. *Int. J. Environ. Res. Public Health* **2021**, *18*, 3902. [CrossRef] [PubMed]
7. Toselli, S.; Marini, E.; Maietta Latessa, P.; Benedetti, L.; Campa, F. Maturity Related Differences in Body Composition Assessed by Classic and Specific Bioimpedance Vector Analysis among Male Elite Youth Soccer Players. *Int. J. Environ. Res. Public Health* **2020**, *17*, 729. [CrossRef]
8. García-Hermoso, A.; Izquierdo, M.; Alonso-Martínez, A.M.; Faigenbaum, A.; Olloquequi, J.; Ramírez-Vélez, R. Association between Exercise-Induced Changes in Cardiorespiratory Fitness and Adiposity among Overweight and Obese Youth: A Meta-Analysis and Meta-Regression Analysis. *Children* **2020**, *7*, 147. [CrossRef]
9. Chulvi-Medrano, I.; Pombo, M.; Saavedra-García, M.Á.; Rebullido, T.R.; Faigenbaum, A.D. A 47-Year Comparison of Lower Body Muscular Power in Spanish Boys: A Short Report. *J. Funct. Morphol. Kinesiol.* **2020**, *5*, 64. [CrossRef]
10. Campa, F.; Greco, G. Special Issue "Growth, Somatic Maturation and Their Impact on Physical Health and Sports Performance". Available online: https://www.mdpi.com/journal/ijerph/special_issues/GSMPPS (accessed on 17 January 2022).
11. Silva, A.F.; Alvurdu, S.; Akyildiz, Z.; Badicu, G.; Greco, G.; Clemente, F.M. Variations of the Locomotor Profile, Sprinting, Change-of-Direction, and Jumping Performances in Youth Soccer Players: Interactions between Playing Positions and Age-Groups. *Int. J. Environ. Res. Public Health* **2022**, *19*, 998. [CrossRef]

12. Ivanović, J.; Kukić, F.; Greco, G.; Koropanovski, N.; Jakovljević, S.; Dopsaj, M. Specific Physical Ability Prediction in Youth Basketball Players According to Playing Position. *Int. J. Environ. Res. Public Health* **2022**, *19*, 977. [CrossRef]
13. Ha, S.; Jeong, H.S.; Park, S.-K.; Lee, S.Y. Can Neurocognitive Function Predict Lower Extremity Injuries in Male Collegiate Athletes? *Int. J. Environ. Res. Public Health* **2020**, *17*, 9061. [CrossRef] [PubMed]
14. Africa, E.; Stryp, O.V.; Musálek, M. The Influence of Cultural Experiences on the Associations between Socio-Economic Status and Motor Performance as Well as Body Fat Percentage of Grade One Learners in Cape Town, South Africa. *Int. J. Environ. Res. Public Health* **2022**, *19*, 121. [CrossRef] [PubMed]
15. Athayde, M.S.d.S.; Kons, R.L.; Fukuda, D.H.; Detanico, D. Body Size Measurements and Physical Performance of Youth Female Judo Athletes with Differing Menarcheal Status. *Int. J. Environ. Res. Public Health* **2021**, *18*, 2829. [CrossRef] [PubMed]
16. Slankamenac, J.; Bjelica, D.; Jaksic, D.; Trivic, T.; Drapsin, M.; Vujkov, S.; Modric, T.; Milosevic, Z.; Drid, P. Somatotype Profiles of Montenegrin Karatekas: An Observational Study. *Int. J. Environ. Res. Public Health* **2021**, *18*, 2914. [CrossRef]
17. Penichet-Tomas, A.; Pueo, B.; Selles-Perez, S.; Jimenez-Olmedo, J.M. Analysis of Anthropometric and Body Composition Profile in Male and Female Traditional Rowers. *Int. J. Environ. Res. Public Health* **2021**, *18*, 7826. [CrossRef]
18. Cattem, M.V.d.O.; Sinforoso, B.T.; Campa, F.; Koury, J.C. Bioimpedance Vector Patterns according to Age and Handgrip Strength in Adolescent Male and Female Athletes. *Int. J. Environ. Res. Public Health* **2021**, *18*, 6069. [CrossRef]
19. Jeong, H.-C.; So, W.-Y. Difficulties of Online Physical Education Classes in Middle and High School and an Efficient Operation Plan to Address Them. *Int. J. Environ. Res. Public Health* **2020**, *17*, 7279. [CrossRef]
20. Guillem, C.M.; Loaiza-Betancur, A.F.; Rebullido, T.R.; Faigenbaum, A.D.; Chulvi-Medrano, I. The Effects of Resistance Training on Blood Pressure in Preadolescents and Adolescents: A Systematic Review and Meta-Analysis. *Int. J. Environ. Res. Public Health* **2020**, *17*, 7900. [CrossRef]
21. Nunes, J.P.; Jacinto, J.L.; Ribeiro, A.S.; Mayhew, J.L.; Nakamura, M.; Capel, D.M.G.; Santos, L.R.; Santos, L.; Cyrino, E.S.; Aguiar, A.F. Placing Greater Torque at Shorter or Longer Muscle Lengths? Effects of Cable vs. Barbell Preacher Curl Training on Muscular Strength and Hypertrophy in Young Adults. *Int. J. Environ. Res. Public Health* **2020**, *17*, 5859. [CrossRef]
22. Campa, F.; Silva, A.M.; Matias, C.N.; Monteiro, C.P.; Paoli, A.; Nunes, J.P.; Talluri, J.; Lukaski, H.; Toselli, S. Body Water Content and Morphological Characteristics Modify Bioimpedance Vector Patterns in Volleyball, Soccer, and Rugby Players. *Int. J. Environ. Res. Public Health* **2020**, *17*, 6604. [CrossRef] [PubMed]
23. Campa, F.; Toselli, S.; Mazzilli, M.; Gobbo, L.A.; Coratella, G. Assessment of Body Composition in Athletes: A Narrative Review of Available Methods with Special Reference to Quantitative and Qualitative Bioimpedance Analysis. *Nutrients* **2021**, *13*, 1620. [CrossRef] [PubMed]
24. Till, K.; Scantlebury, S.; Jones, B. Anthropometric and Physical Qualities of Elite Male Youth Rugby League Players. *Sports Med.* **2017**, *47*, 2171–2186. [CrossRef] [PubMed]

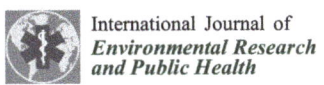

Article

Variations of the Locomotor Profile, Sprinting, Change-of-Direction, and Jumping Performances in Youth Soccer Players: Interactions between Playing Positions and Age-Groups

Ana Filipa Silva [1,2,3], Sümer Alvurdu [4], Zeki Akyildiz [4], Georgian Badicu [5], Gianpiero Greco [6,*] and Filipe Manuel Clemente [1,2,7]

1. Escola Superior Desporto e Lazer, Instituto Politécnico de Viana do Castelo, Rua Escola Industrial e Comercial de Nun'Álvares, 4900-347 Viana do Castelo, Portugal; anafilsilva@gmail.com (A.F.S.); filipe.clemente5@gmail.com (F.M.C.)
2. The Research Centre in Sports Sciences, Health Sciences and Human Development (CIDESD), 5001-801 Vila Real, Portugal
3. Research Center in Sports Performance, Recreation, Innovation and Technology (SPRINT), 4960-320 Melgaço, Portugal
4. Faculty of Sport Sciences, Gazi University, Ankara 06700, Turkey; sumeralvurdu@gazi.edu.tr (S.A.); zekiakyldz@hotmail.com (Z.A.)
5. Department of Physical Education and Special Motricity, Faculty of Physical Education and Mountain Sports, Transilvania University of Brașov, 500068 Brașov, Romania; georgian.badicu@unitbv.ro
6. Department of Basic Medical Sciences, Neuroscience and Sense Organs, University of Study of Bari, 70121 Bari, Italy
7. Instituto de Telecomunicações, Delegação da Covilhã, 1049-001 Lisboa, Portugal
* Correspondence: gianpierogreco.phd@yahoo.com

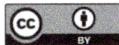

Abstract: The purpose of this study was two-fold: (i) analyze the variations of locomotor profile, sprinting, change-of-direction (COD) and jumping performances between different youth age-groups; and (ii) test the interaction effect of athletic performance with playing positions. A cross-sectional study design was followed. A total of 124 youth soccer players from five age-groups were analyzed once in a time. Players were classified based on their typical playing position. The following measures were obtained: (i) body composition (fat mass); (ii) jump height (measured in the countermovement jump; CMJ); (iii) sprinting time at 5-, 10-, 15-, 20-, 25- and 30-m; (iv) maximal sprint speed (measured in the best split time; MSS); (v) COD asymmetry index percentage); (vi) final velocity at 30-15 Intermittent Fitness Test (V_{IFT}); and (vii) anaerobic speed reserve (ASR = MSS − V_{IFT}). A two-way ANOVA was used for establishing the interactions between age-groups and playing positions. Significant differences were found between age-groups in CMJ ($p < 0.001$), 5-m ($p < 0.001$), 10-m ($p < 0.001$), 15-m ($p < 0.001$), 20-m ($p < 0.001$), 25-m ($p < 0.001$), 30-m ($p < 0.001$), V_{IFT} ($p < 0.001$), ASR ($p = 0.003$), MSS ($p < 0.001$), COD ($p < 0.001$). Regarding variations between playing positions no significant differences were found. In conclusion, it was found that the main factor influencing changes in physical fitness was the age group while playing positions had no influence on the variations in the assessed parameters. In particular, as older the age group, as better was in jumping, sprinting, COD, and locomotor profile.

Keywords: football; athletic performance; physical fitness; exercise test

1. Introduction

The soccer match requires from the players a well and multilateral developed physical fitness [1,2]. In fact, considering that the soccer game is an intermittent exercise with a mix of bioenergetic demands it is expectable to observe in players a good ability to sustain prolonged efforts and, at the same time, the availability to intensify the actions in more powerful movements [3,4]. Looking into the physical demands of the match, most of the time is spent in low-to-moderate running intensities [5,6], although the percentage of time spent in high intensity running or sprinting has been increasing over the years for the same total distance covered [7–9]. Thus, the match is becoming more intense requiring from the players a superior level of conditioning to sustain such intensifications [10,11]. Although ultimate performance in soccer is multifactorial, some of the critical events (e.g., goal-oriented events) are closely related to high-intensity running demands [5,6]. Thus, holding a good physical fitness can be a support for the ultimate performance [12,13].

Characterizing physical fitness is now a well-implemented practice in soccer [14]. The battery of tests is commonly used in different periods of the seasons helping strength and conditioning coaches to individualize the training process, identify the status of the players and observe the evolution trends of the players over the season [14]. Moreover, in the particular case of youth, longitudinal observations/assessments also allow to identify talents across the time. Although talent identification is a complex and multidimensional process [15,16], using physical fitness parameters as part of talent identification processes is still prevalent [17]. As example, using physical fitness batteries allows to identify that in some age groups the taller, heavier and more physical advanced players are those with higher levels [18,19]. Although these facts not being exclusively related to the ultimate players' selection and transition for professional careers, tracking players over time can provide some additional information about which expectations coaches should have regarding their players and the evolution trends of the players over time and also determine how players can cope with match intensity [20].

For the case of physical fitness, it seems that the breaking point of 14/15 years old is the one in which change-of-direction (COD), linear sprint, standing long jump and aerobic capacity tests makes more sense are more sensitive to age-related changes in functional characteristics [21,22]. Moreover, testing batteries consisting in either vertical/horizontal jumps, sprinting and COD and aerobic fitness seems to be sensitive enough to distinguish between different youth age groups [23]. Interestingly, the most common tests as countermovement jump (CMJ), 5-0-5 (COD test), 10- to 20-m linear sprint test or standing broad jump are proven to be highly reliable and valid for youth soccer players [24].

Although the above-mentioned tests present a good consensus about the usability for practice, some other tests can be used directly helping coaches to prescribe the training process and classify the youth players. As example, the 30-15 Intermittent Fitness Test (30-15IFT) has been used for standardize the training intensity while applying high-intensity interval training [25]. Moreover, combining the final velocity at 30-15IFT and the maximal sprint speed (MSS) it is possible to obtain the anaerobic speed reserve (ASR) of the players and classify them into their locomotor profile (e.g., speed, hybrid, and endurance) [26].

Observing positive changes of physical fitness across the age-groups seems to be expectable [27]. However, in the context of soccer, playing positions seems to play an important role to differentiate players [27]. In a study conducted in a large sample of 744 youth players it was observed that after the age of 15, the attackers tends to be more explosive, the fastest and more agile players [28]. This tendency of observing greater differences in the later stages of development programs was also confirmed in a study conducted in 465 youth players [29].

The relevance of characterization the progression of physical fitness across age-groups, while in interaction with playing position seems to be obvious. This may help coaches to better specify and individualize the training process and classify the players based on their abilities to sustain and maintain match intensities. Therefore, the purpose of this study was two-fold: (i) analyze the variations of locomotor profile, sprinting, change-of-direction (COD) and jumping performances between different youth age-groups; and (ii) test the interaction effect of athletic performance with playing positions.

2. Materials and Methods

2.1. Study Design

This study followed a cross-sectional design. Players were recruited in the same team and no randomization was made. Age groups of 19 and 17 years old were assessed on 31 August 2021 and 1 September 2021. Age groups of 16 and 15 years old were assessed on 1 September 2021 and 2 September 2021. Age group of 14 years old was assessed on 2 September 2021 and 3 September 2021. The study begun after 3 weeks of the beginning of the season. As context, 24 number of training sessions were performed, and 3 friendly matches occurred before the study begun.

2.2. Participants

The G*Power (version 3.1.) was used to calculate the a priori sample size. For a partial eta squared of 0.6 (medium effect size), a $p = 0.05$, power of 0.80, numerator df of 8 and number of groups of 10, the suggested total sample size was 20. A total of 124 young male elite male soccer players from U15 ($n = 29$), U16 ($n = 30$), U17 ($n = 27$), U18 ($n = 25$), and U19 ($n = 12$) teams were recruited voluntarily to participate in the study. All these players were regularly involved in two training sessions a week (90 min per session) with participation in one match at the weekend. Players and their guardians were informed about the study design and protocol. After being informed for potential risks of the study, guardians signed informed consent forms. This study followed the ethical principles of the Helsinki Declaration for human research. A local ethics committee also approved the protocol. Inclusion criteria for the participants were (i) being an active player with at least three years license, (ii) no history of any injuries during the previous two months, (iii) participating %85 of the training during the study period.

2.3. Testing Procedures

The study were carried out in two different days, separated by a minimum of 48 h. On the first day, anthropometric assessment (height, body mass and body fat percentage), and performance tests (vertical jumping, sprinting and change-of-direction ability) were applied respectively. The assessments of the first day occurred at 2:00 p.m. of the day, in a room conditioned at 24 degrees Celsius and 52% relative humidity. Second day, 30-15 IFT test were performed to evaluate the final velocity (V_{IFT}) and anaerobic speed reserve (ASR) in the following conditions: 03:00 p.m., 19 degrees Celsius and 49% relative humidity. Players were familiarized with all test at the previous seasons. All performance tests were conducted on a synthetic turf field (where the players train and compete) after a standardized FIFA 11+ warm-up protocol [30] (ref).

2.3.1. Anthropometry

A measuring tape (SECA 206, Hamburg, Germany) and a digital scale (SECA 874, Hamburg, Germany) with an accuracy of 0.1 kg were used to measure the height and body mass of the participants. Body fat percentage was evaluated with 4-site skinfold measurement (biceps, triceps, iliac crest and subscapular) according to the Durnin–Womersley formula [31]. At least two measurements were taken from each athlete and if there was more than 5 percent difference between the two measurements, the third measurement was taken.

2.3.2. Jumping Performance

Countermovement Jump (CMJ) was used to evaluate participants' jumping performances with Optojump optical measurement system (OptojumpNext, Microgate, Bolzano, Italy). The participants performed three vertical attempts with 2 min recovery and the best attempt was used for the analyses. During the attempt, the participants were asked to jump keeping their hands on the hips and without bending the legs from take-off and landing phase.

2.3.3. Sprinting

The 30 m linear sprint test with 5 m splits (5-, 10-, 15-, 20-, 25-, 30) were measured using the electronic timing gates system (Smartspeed, Fusion Sport, QLD, Australia). The timing gates were positioned at 1.2 m height of the floor. Players positioned 0.5 m far from the first timing gate and were encouraged to sprint at maximum speed and were given to two attempts with three minutes of recovery to prevent fatigue. Players took their preferred foot one step forward before the start and no signal was given. They started in split position, and always with the same preferred leg. The best sprinting time (lower value) was used for the analysis.

2.3.4. Maximal Speed Sprint

The MSS was estimated using the average time over the last 10- and 5-m splits of a 30-m sprint test. A previous study revealed that using both 10- and 5-m splits of a 30-m sprint test while using timing gates can be reliability and present a high level of agreement with the MSS estimated using a gold-standard radar gun [32].

2.3.5. Change-of-Direction Ability

The Arrowhead agility test was used for the participants' COD ability. Electronic timing gates system (Smartspeed, Fusion Sport, QLD, Australia) positioned at the start line with a height of 1.2 m starting from the floor. The participant positioned 0.50 m from the timing gate and sprinted from the start line to the middle marker (A), turned to the left or right side to sprint around the marker (B), sprinted around the top marker (C) and sprinted back through the timing gate to finish the test [33]. Athletes were asked to use their right leg when they turned left, and their left leg when they turned right as breaking legs. The test was performed for left and right sides with four randomized attempts separated by at least three minutes of recovery. The best attempts of each side was recorded for analysis.

The asymmetry index was calculated according to the following formula [34]:

Asymmetry Index percentage (AI%):

$$AI\% = [(COD\ time_{Dominant} - COD\ time_{Non\text{-}dominant})/COD\ time_{Dominant}] \times 100$$

2.3.6. Velocity at 30-15 IFT and Anaerobic Speed Reserve

The 30-15IFT was performed by the participants according to the protocol developed by Buchheit [25]. The tests consist in perform 30 s shuttle runs interspersed with 15 s of passive recovery. The test starts with a velocity of 8 km/h. The speed increases by 0.5 km/h after each stage (30-s). Every time the player was unable to reach the line with the pace imposed by the audio beep, was marked. After failing three consecutive times, the final velocity achieved correctly was considered for further analysis. The last completed stage was used to determine the final velocity (V_{IFT}) and anaerobic speed reserve was calculated as the difference between MSS and V_{IFT} with the following equation [35]:

$$ASR\ (km/h) = MSS - V_{IFT}$$

2.4. Statistical Analyses

Shapiro-Wilk and Levene tests were used to test the assumption of normality and homoscedasticity, respectively. Both, normality and homogeneity were confirmed with $p > 0.05$. Then, Bonferroni homoscedasticity and Two-way ANOVA were used, respectively. The Two Way ANOVA with Bonferroni post hoc test was used to compare player positions and ages. All statistical analyses were performed using RStudio Version: 2021.09.1 + 372. Statistics at a significance level of $p < 0.05$. The following scale was used to classify the effect sizes (ES) of the tests: small, 0.2–0.49; moderate, 0.50–0.79; large, 0.80–1. Partial eta-squared was used ANOVA and Cohen D to pairwise comparisons.

3. Results

Two-way ANOVA tested interactions between age-groups and playing positions. No significant interactions were found on height ($p = 0.031$; $\eta^2_p = 0.235$), body mass ($p = 0.235$; $\eta^2_p = 0.171$), body fat ($p = 0.635$; $\eta^2_p = 0.121$), CMJ ($p = 0.027$; $\eta^2_p = 0.239$), 5-m ($p = 0.412$; $\eta^2_p = 0.146$), 10-m ($p = 0.490$; $\eta^2_p = 0.137$), 15-m ($p = 0.582$; $\eta^2_p = 0.127$), 20-m ($p = 0.464$; $\eta^2_p = 0.140$), 25-m ($p = 0.178$; $\eta^2_p = 0.182$) and 30-m ($p = 0.252$; $\eta^2_p = 0.168$), MSS ($p = 0.388$; $\eta^2_p = 0.149$), VITF ($p = 0.166$; $\eta^2_p = 0.184$), ASR ($p = 0.441$; $\eta^2_p = 0.143$), COD right ($p = 0.159$; $\eta^2_p = 0.186$), COD left ($p = 0.662$; $\eta^2_p = 0.118$), and COD-AI% ($p = 0.598$; $\eta^2_p = 0.125$).

One-way ANOVA tested the variations of physical fitness measures between age-groups. Descriptive statistics can be found in the Table 1 (anthropometrics) and Table 2 (physical fitness). Results revealed that the age group of 14 years old was significantly smaller and lighter ($p < 0.05$) than the remaining age groups. No other significant differences were found regarding anthropometric outcomes.

Table 1. Descriptive statistics (mean and standard deviation) for the anthropometric outcomes between age-groups.

Measure	14 yo (N = 29)	15 yo (N = 30)	16 yo (N = 27)	17 yo (N = 25)	18 yo (N = 12)	p	ES
Height (cm)	167.65 ± 7.02 [b,c,d,e]	174.80 ± 4.70 [a]	176.14 ± 6.63 [a]	175.48 ± 7.04 [a]	177.16 ± 4.89 [a]	0.001	0.243
BM (kg)	57.43 ± 7.90 [b,c,d,e]	64.54 ± 5.79 [a]	65.82 ± 5.96 [a]	67.78 ± 6.52 [a]	69.32 ± 5.77 [a]	0.001	0.288
BF (kg)	8.94 ± 2.82	7.82 ± 1.69	8.14 ± 1.81	9.06 ± 2.30	8.45 ± 1.93	0.173	0.052

Yo: years old; BM: body mass; Body fat: BF; significant different from 14 yo [a]; 15 yo [b]; 16 yo [c]; 17 yo [d]; and 18 yo [e] at $p < 0.05$.

Results from Table 2 revealed that the younger age group (under-14) had significant smaller values of CMJ ($p < 0.05$), was significantly slower at 5-, 10-, 15-, 20-, 25- and 30-m distances and COD right ($p < 0.05$), and had significant smaller MSS, VIFT, and ASR ($p < 0.05$) than the remaining age-groups.

Table 2. Descriptive statistics (mean and standard deviation) for the physical fitness outcomes between age-groups.

Measure	14 yo (N = 29)	15 yo (N = 30)	16 yo (N = 27)	17 yo (N = 25)	18 yo (N = 12)	p	ES
CMJ (cm)	36.95 ± 4.70 [c,d]	37.96 ± 4.49 [c]	42.08 ± 7.07 [a,b]	42.02 ± 6.04 [a]	41.04 ± 4.92	0.001	0.145
5-m (s)	1.39 ± 0.10 [b,c,d,e]	1.29 ± 0.1 [a,d,e]	1.29 ± 0.09 [a,d,e]	1.10 ± 0.11 [a,b,d,e]	1.10 ± 0.08 [a,b,c]	0.001	0.517
10-m (s)	2.14 ± 0.11 [b,c,d,e]	2.04 ± 0.11 [a,d,e]	2.04 ± 0.09 [a,d,e]	1.81 ± 0.14 [a,b,c]	1.79 ± 0.10 [a,b,c]	0.001	0.562
15-m (s)	2.88 ± 0.14 [b,c,d,e]	2.70 ± 0.15 [a,d,e]	2.68 ± 0.11 [a,d,e]	2.44 ± 0.19 [a,b,c]	2.41 ± 0.12 [a,b,c]	0.001	0.566
20-m (s)	3.57 ± 0.16 [b,c,d,e]	3.38 ± 0.16 [a,d,e]	3.32 ± 0.14 [a,d,e]	3.07 ± 0.20 [a,b,c,e]	3.03 ± 0.12 [a,b,c]	0.001	0.573
25-m (s)	4.21 ± 0.19 [b,c,d,e]	4.06 ± 0.17 [a,d,e]	3.97 ± 0.16 [a,d,e]	3.68 ± 0.22 [a,b,c]	3.63 ± 0.14 [a,b,c]	0.001	0.571
30-m (s)	4.86 ± 0.22 [b,c,d,e]	4.65 ± 0.20 [a,d,e]	4.54 ± 0.18	4.24 ± 0.23 [a,d,e]	4.21 ± 0.16 [a,b,c]	0.001	0.570
MSS (km/h)	28.60 ± 1.69 [b,c,d,e]	30.80 ± 2.72 [a]	31.85 ± 2.75 [a]	32.24 ± 2.21 [a]	32.01 ± 1.88 [a]	0.001	0.268
V_{IFT} (km/h)	17.44 ± 1.49 [c,d,e]	18.35 ± 1.19	18.44 ± 1.08 [a]	18.80 ± 1.24 [a]	19.54 ± 0.89 [a]	0.001	0.203
ASR (km/h)	11.15 ± 2.05 [c,d]	12.45 ± 3.04	13.41 ± 2.80 [a]	13.44 ± 2.28 [a]	12.47 ± 2.30	0.007	0.111
COD right (s)	9.27 ± 0.25 [b,c,d,e]	9.0 ± 0.36 [a,d,e]	8.90 ± 0.29 [a]	8.71 ± 0.22 [a,b]	8.70 ± 0.14 [a,b]	0.001	0.338

Table 2. Cont.

Measure	14 yo (N = 29)	15 yo (N = 30)	16 yo (N = 27)	17 yo (N = 25)	18 yo (N = 12)	p	ES
COD left (s)	9.20 ± 0.29	8.97 ± 0.31	8.88 ± 0.29	8.76 ± 0.25	8.67 ± 0.18	0.001	0.228
COD–AI%	−1.94 ± 1.19	−2.64 ± 2.50[c]	−1.34 ± 0.76[b]	−1.74 ± 0.89	−1.64 ± 1.35	0.029	0.086

Yo: years old; CMJ: countermovement jump; MSS: maximal sprint speed; VIFT: final velocity at 30-15 Intermittent fitness test; ASR: anaerobic speed reserve; COD: change-of-direction; COD-AI%: Change-of-Direction Asymmetry Index percentage; significant different from 14 yo [a]; 15 yo [b]; 16 yo [c]; 17 yo [d]; and 18 yo [e] at $p < 0.05$.

One-way ANOVA tested the variations of physical fitness measures between playing positions. Descriptive statistics can be found in the Table 3 (anthropometrics) and Table 4 (physical fitness. Results from Table 3 revealed that central defenders and forwards were significantly taller and heavier ($p < 0.05$) than the remaining positions. No significant differences were found regarding body fat.

Table 3. Descriptive statistics (mean and standard deviation) for the athropometric outcomes between playing positions.

Measure	CD (N = 26)	CM (N = 33)	ED (N = 26)	EM (N = 19)	F (N = 19)	p	ES
Height (cm)	178.73 ± 5.04 [b,c,d]	172.12 ± 7.76 [a,e]	170.73 ± 5.42 [a,e]	170.42 ± 3.97 [a,e]	177.42 ± 7.55 [b,c,d]	0.001	0.235
BM (kg)	68.61 ± 4.61 [b,c,d]	62.73 ± 8.85 [a]	62.19 ± 7.42 [a]	61.46 ± 5.03 [a]	66.64 ± 8.36	0.002	0.132
BF (kg)	8.34 ± 2.30	8.54 ± 2.16	8.80 ± 2.44	7.94 ± 1.75	8.59 ± 2.30	0.772	0.015

CD: central defender; ED: external defender; CM: central midfielder; EM: external midfielder; F: forward; BM: body mass; Body fat: BF; significant different from CD [a]; CM [b]; ED [c]; EM [d]; and F [e] at $p < 0.05$

Results from Table 4 revealed no significant differences between playing positions regarding the physical fitness outcomes.

Table 4. Descriptive statistics (mean and standard deviation) for the physical fitness outcomes between playing positions.

Measure	CD (N = 26)	CM (N = 33)	ED (N = 26)	EM (N = 19)	F (N = 19)	p	ES
CMJ (cm)	38.88 ± 5.76	38.68 ± 4.58	39.30 ± 5.81	42.31 ± 7.87	40.88 ± 5.72	0.195	0.050
5-m (s)	1.27 ± 0.14	1.25 ± 0.14	1.27 ± 0.13	1.23 ± 0.18	1.25 ± 0.16	0.861	0.011
10-m (s)	2 ± 0.15	2 ± 0.17	2.02 ± 0.14	1.95 ± 0.21	1.98 ± 0.21	0.714	0.018
15-m (s)	2.68 ± 0.20	2.68 ± 0.22	2.67 ± 0.19	2.59 ± 0.26	2.63 ± 0.25	0.688	0.019
20-m (s)	3.34 ± 0.21	3.34 ± 0.25	3.32 ± 0.21	3.23 ± 0.30	3.30 ± 0.27	0.594	0.023
25-m (s)	3.99 ± 0.23	3.98 ± 0.29	3.97 ± 0.23	3.87 ± 0.33	3.94 ± 0.31	0.665	0.020
30-m (s)	4.58 ± 0.25	4.58 ± 0.33	4.56 ± 0.28	4.46 ± 0.37	4.54 ± 0.35	0.699	0.018
MSS (km/h)	30.76 ± 2.50	30.52 ± 0.64	31.18 ± 2.98	31.34 ± 2.61	31.06 ± 2.87	0.820	0.013
V_{IFT} (km/h)	18.09 ± 1.34	18.42 ± 1.50	18.55 ± 1.13	18.71 ± 1.05	18.02 ± 1.64	0.411	0.033
ASR (km/h)	12.67 ± 2.57	12.10 ± 2.60	12.63 ± 3.16	12.63 ± 2.34	13.03 ± 2.66	0.806	0.013
COD right (s)	8.91 ± 0.36	9 ± 0.32	8.93 ± 0.34	8.87 ± 0.30	9 ± 0.38	0.591	0.023
COD left (s)	8.91 ± 0.31	8.99 ± 0.34	8.94 ± 0.35	8.86 ± 0.33	8.93 ± 0.32	0.741	0.016
COD–AI%	−1.90 ± 1.97	−1.83 ± 1.35	−2.19 ± 1.99	−1.82 ± 1.05	−1.76 ± 1.18	0.890	0.009

CD: central defender; ED: external defender; CM: central midfielder; EM: external midfielder; F: forward; BM: body mass; Body fat: BF; CMJ: countermovement jump; MSS: maximal sprint speed; VIFT: final velocity at 30-15 Intermittent fitness test; ASR: anaerobic speed reserve; COD: change-of-direction; COD-AI%: Change-of-Direction Asymmetry Index percentage; significant different from CD; CM; ED; EM; and F at $p < 0.05$.

In Figure 1, descriptive plots for anthropometry, CMJ, 5-m and 10-m were presented. Although no significant differences between playing positions, it is evident a significant difference of the younger age-group for being smaller and lighter than the remaining age groups.

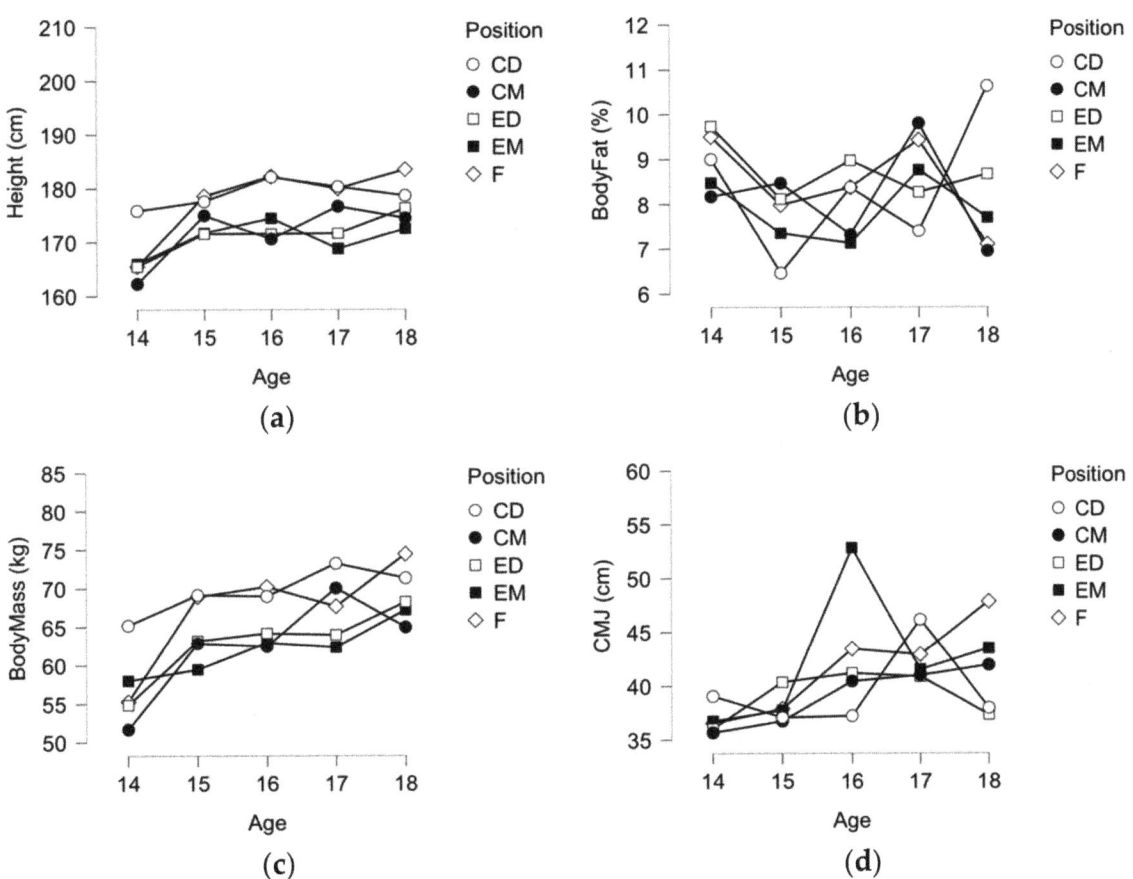

Figure 1. Descriptive plots for (a) height (cm); (b) body fat (%), (c) body mass (kg); and (d) CMJ (cm).

In Figure 2, descriptive plots for 15 m, 20 m, 25 m, 30 m, Maximum Speed, and ASR were presented. It seems evident a significant trend for being faster as older as players are (independently of the distance considered in the sprint test). Moreover, maximal speed sprint and anaerobic speed reserve also increase as players are older.

In Figure 3, descriptive plots for COD Right, COD Left, Asymmetry Index, COD-AI%, and VIFT were presented. As older players are, the better COD performance they get. Although no significant differences can be observed in the asymmetry index with exception of the pair of 15 and 16 years old. The VIFT is also significantly rising with the increase of age groups.

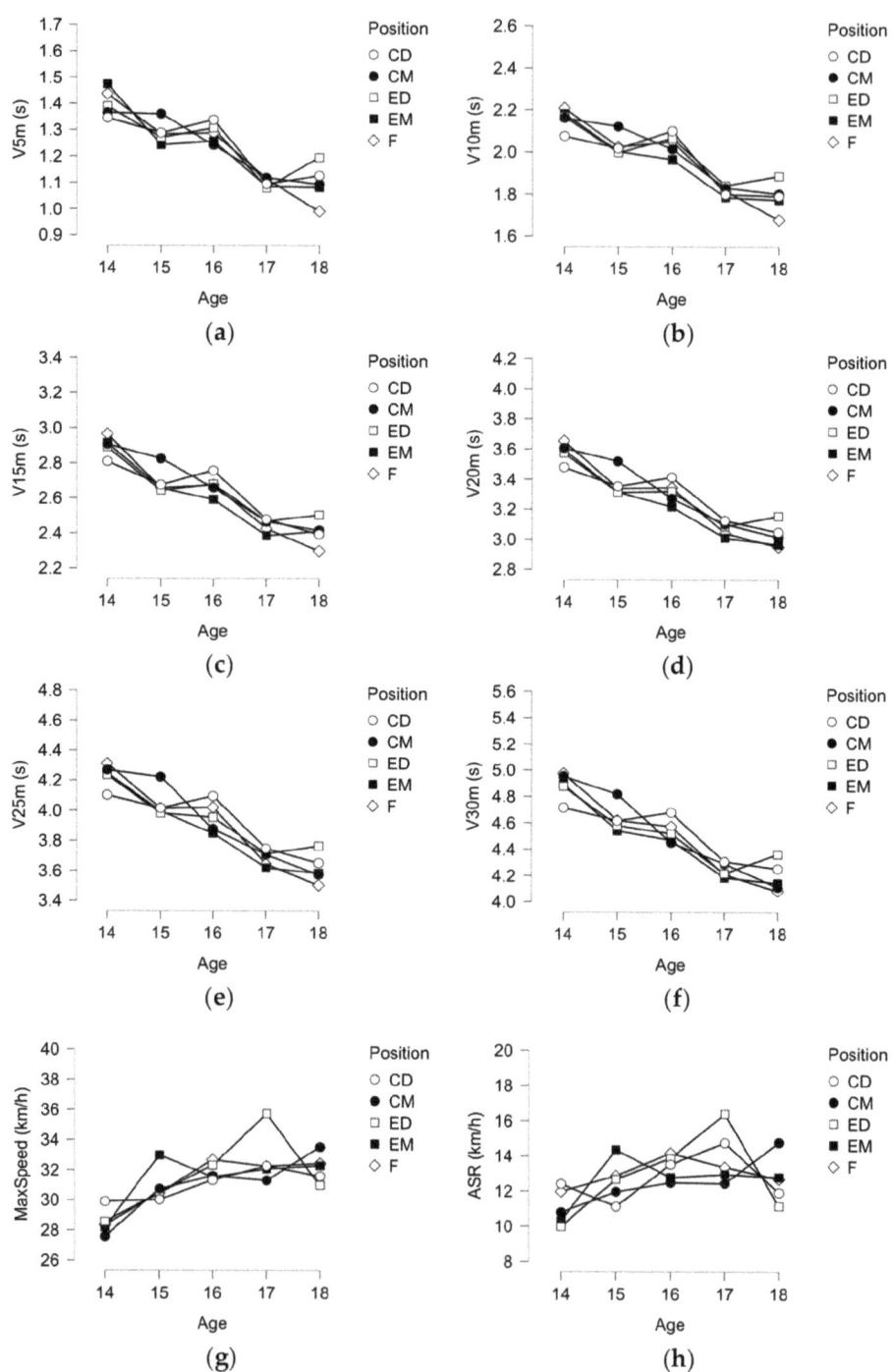

Figure 2. Descriptive plots for (**a**) 5-m; (**b**) 10-m; (**c**) 15-m; (**d**) 20-m; (**e**) 25-m; and (**f**) 30-m sprint time (s) and (**g**) maximal speed sprint (km/h); and (**h**) anaerobic speed reserve (km/h).

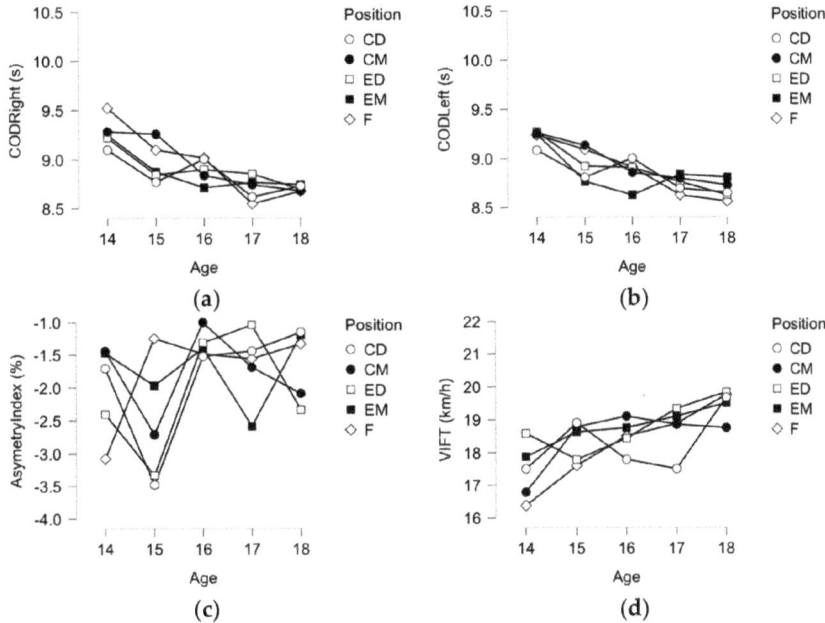

Figure 3. Descriptive plots (**a**) COD right leg (s); (**b**) COD left leg (s); (**c**) asymmetry index percentage (%); and (**d**) VIFT (km/h).

4. Discussion

The current cross-sectional study conducted over 124 youth soccer players revealed that age groups play a significant effect on physical fitness while playing positions were not capable to determine variations in physical fitness. Considering that significant changes in physical fitness were found between age groups, it was also observed that the older the groups, the better the results. Therefore, from 14 to 18 years old, the players turn taller, heavier, faster, while jumping higher and having a greater locomotor profile to sustain the efforts.

4.1. Age Group Comparisons

The normal growth patterns were found in the current research, namely considering the progressive increase of height and body mass until the last stage of youth [36,37]. Thus, the older the player is in youth soccer, the taller and heavier is. Such an evidence is confirmed in previous studies comparing different age groups withing the period of growth [38,39]. Interestingly, in the contrary to a possible expectation of observing an improvement in body fat levels [39,40], no significant differences were found across the age-groups in the current study. One of the causes could be the small body fat levels observed in the current study (mean values were stable around 8% over the ages) which is low, mainly in comparison to the studies reporting body fat in youth soccer players which presented values between 7 and 11% [36]. Also, in the opposite to expected [28,41], no significant differences were found in anthropometric and body composition data between playing positions. Although the current sample does not include goalkeepers (which is one of the positions favorable to be taller than remaining) [42], it would be expectable to observe significant variations between the remaining positions. As average (since interactions with age was not found), playing positions varied from 170 to 180 cm, while body mass between 60 and 70 kg. Although variations were observed, no significances were found, which may indicate that the tendency for selecting players based on playing position may not be too much implemented in the context of this group of players (considering that all of them belong to the same club).

In the current study it was found that as older the players as faster they are. Considering the different measures related with sprinting performance (e.g., 5-, 10-, 15-, 20-, 25-, 30-, and MSS) and COD performance it was observed a progressive and significant improvement until reach the final stage of youth soccer (i.e., 18 years old). These tendencies are in line with previous reports for youth soccer players [43,44]. Some possible explanations can be related with the growth and maturation that plays an important role in the muscular adaptation and neural drive, and bioenergetics to sustain MSS in late puberty [45]. Lower limb power observed in the improvements of CMJ over the age groups considered can possibly explain those advantages in neural and muscular adaptations over age. Although huge differences in the determinants that explains different linear sprint distances and COD, it was interesting to observe that older were always better in any of sprint test distances, COD measures and CMJ.

Therefore, it can be argued that older tends to accelerate better (possibly explained by the greater concentric force and power which was possible observed by the increases in CMJ performance over the age-groups) [46], achieve higher velocities (possible explained by a greater eccentric force, vertical force and power) [47] and can decelerate and accelerate better due to the better neuromuscular properties [48] developed in accordance to the training process, and normal increase in muscular adaptation and neural drive. In, fact, considering that older can reach a greater MSS than younger [49], it is expectable that such a stimulus in match and training can play an important role in the development of sprinting and COD performance since achieving peak speed is an effective way of improve it [50,51]. However, as major factors can be listed maturation and the related neural function, multi-joint coordination, muscle stiffness, and changes in muscle architecture [52].

In the current study it was also found that locomotor profile determined by ASR and VIFT followed the trend of the older, the better. Considering that locomotor profile is highly associated with aerobic fitness, it is expectable to observe natural and progressive increases after the maturational peak until reach the 16 years old in males [52,53]. These changes and increases are potentially explained by changes occurring in central mechanisms namely considering the increase of heart, lungs, muscles and blood volume [54,55]. Naturally, other factors as hormonal or enzymatic can be also important for ultimately improving the progressive improvement of aerobic fitness during the youth stages [56]. Thus, this can justify improvements in aerobic power as well as in the maximal aerobic speed which may justifies improvements in V_{IFT} [57]. Considering that VIFT is justified by different measures including aerobic fitness, change-of-direction or lower limb power, and taking in consideration that the older, the better in these levels, VIFT tends to be improved also across the age-groups. Moreover, considering that anaerobic systems is improved after peak maturation [58,59], it is also expectable to assist to an improvement of ASR as well [60].

4.2. Playing Position Comparisons

One of the common trends observed over the current results were the absence of playing position effect on the physical fitness variation of youth soccer players. This is not in line with most of studies conducted in soccer, mainly those conducted in later stages of youth formation [28,29]. Possibly, a better fitness level observed can mask positional differences that traditionally occur in players based on the specificity of the training process and match demands. Future research should focus in analyze if a proper training process can mitigate differences between playing positions, or on the other side, a training process based on the average and not individuality can also decrease differences between playing positions.

4.3. Study Limitations, Future Research and Practical Implications

The fact of the study has been conducted in only one club can be a source of bias, like many other cross-sectional studies conducted in this field of research. Observational analytic studies to determine differences between age groups and playing positions should be made in the future with more than one context and determine how the context can play a role or not in the evidence collected. Despite the limitation, this study was conducted in 124 players which is substantial and allows a sample enough to confirm the evidence. As practical implications, this study may suggest that as older, as better. Thus, with the progression in age, a more focused stimulus can be provided on the physical fitness, and possible more individualization and specificity of training can occur to ensure the adjustment to the position specificities of the game.

5. Conclusions

This study revealed that the older, the better in terms of physical fitness in youth soccer players. Considering the age-groups included (14 to 18 years old), improvements in locomotor profile, sprinting, change-of-direction, and jumping performance were significant and obvious. Younger players were significantly smaller and lighter, while were significantly slower, jump smaller and had less maximal speed sprint, anaerobic speed reserve and V_{IFT}. Although this evidence was not found significant interactions of age-group with playing positions and, additionally, playing positions did not differentiate athletes.

Author Contributions: Conceptualization, A.F.S., Z.A. and F.M.C.; methodology, S.A.; formal analysis, Z.A.; data curation, S.A.; writing—original draft preparation, A.F.S., S.A., Z.A., G.B., G.G. and F.M.C.; writing—review and editing, A.F.S., S.A., Z.A., G.B., G.G. and F.M.C. All authors have read and agreed to the published version of the manuscript.

Funding: This work is funded by Fundação para a Ciência e Tecnologia/ Ministério da Ciência, Tecnologia e Ensino Superior through national funds and when applicable co-funded EU funds under the project UIDB/50008/2020.

Institutional Review Board Statement: The study was conducted according to the guidelines of the Declaration of Helsinki, and approved by the Ethics Committee of University of Gazi (approval: GAZI/2021).

Informed Consent Statement: Informed consent was obtained from all subjects involved in the study.

Data Availability Statement: Raw data of this article are available upon request to corresponding author.

Conflicts of Interest: The authors declare no conflict of interest.

References

1. Drust, B.; Atkinson, G.; Reilly, T. Future Perspectives in the Evaluation of the Physiological Demands of Soccer. *Sport Med.* **2007**, *37*, 783–805. [CrossRef] [PubMed]
2. Mohr, M.; Krustrup, P.; Bangsbo, J. Fatigue in soccer: A brief review. *J. Sports Sci.* **2005**, *23*, 593–599. [CrossRef] [PubMed]
3. Dolci, F.; Hart, N.H.; Kilding, A.E.; Chivers, P.; Piggott, B.; Spiteri, T. Physical and Energetic Demand of Soccer: A Brief Review. *Strength Cond. J.* **2020**, *42*, 70–77. [CrossRef]
4. Stolen, T.; Chamari, K.; Castagna, C.; Wisloff, U. Physiology of soccer: An update. *Sport Med.* **2005**, *35*, 501–536. [CrossRef]
5. Andrzejewski, M.; Chmura, J.; Pluta, B.; Strzelczyk, R.; Kasprzak, A. Analysis of Sprinting Activities of Professional Soccer Players. *J. Strength Cond. Res.* **2013**, *27*, 2134–2140. [CrossRef]
6. Faude, O.; Koch, T.; Meyer, T. Straight sprinting is the most frequent action in goal situations in professional football. *J. Sports Sci.* **2012**, *30*, 625–631. [CrossRef] [PubMed]
7. Bradley, P.S.; Archer, D.T.; Hogg, B.; Schuth, G.; Bush, M.; Carling, C.; Barnes, C. Tier-specific evolution of match performance characteristics in the English Premier League: It's getting tougher at the top. *J. Sports Sci.* **2016**, *34*, 980–987. [CrossRef]
8. Bush, M.; Barnes, C.; Archer, D.T.; Hogg, B.; Bradley, P.S. Evolution of match performance parameters for various playing positions in the English Premier League. *Hum. Mov. Sci.* **2015**, *39*, 1–11. [CrossRef] [PubMed]
9. Pons, E.; Ponce-Bordón, J.C.; Díaz-García, J.; Del Campo, R.L.; Resta, R.; Peirau, X.; García-Calvo, T. A longitudinal exploration of match running performance during a football match in the spanish la liga: A four-season study. *Int. J. Environ. Res. Public Health* **2021**, *18*, 1133. [CrossRef]

10. Oliva-Lozano, J.M.; Gómez-Carmona, C.D.; Pino-Ortega, J.; Moreno-Pérez, V.; Rodríguez-Pérez, M.A. Match and Training High Intensity Activity-Demands Profile during a Competitive Mesocycle in Youth Elite Soccer Players. *J. Hum. Kinet.* **2020**, *75*, 195–205. [CrossRef]
11. Duthie, G.M.; Thornton, H.R.; Delaney, J.A.; Connolly, D.R.; Serpiello, F.R. Running Intensities in Elite Youth Soccer by Age and Position. *J. Strength Cond. Res.* **2018**, *32*, 2918–2924. [CrossRef] [PubMed]
12. Krustrup, P.; Mohr, M.; Amstrup, T.; Rysgaard, T.; Johansen, J.; Steensberg, A.; Preben, K.; Bangsbo, J. The Yo-Yo Intermittent Recovery Test: Physiological Response, Reliability, and Validity. *Med. Sci. Sport Exerc.* **2003**, *35*, 697–705. [CrossRef] [PubMed]
13. Krustrup, P.; Mohr, M.; Ellingsgaard, H.; Bangsbo, J.; Ellinsgaard, H.; Bangsbo, J. Physical Demands during an Elite Female Soccer Game: Importance of Training Status. *Med. Sci. Sport Exerc.* **2005**, *37*, 1242–1248. [CrossRef] [PubMed]
14. Turner, A.; Walker, S.; Stembridge, M.; Coneyworth, P.; Reed, G.; Birdsey, L.; Barter, L.; Moody, J. A Testing Battery for the Assessment of Fitness in Soccer Players. *Strength Cond. J.* **2011**, *33*, 29–39. [CrossRef]
15. Sarmento, H.; Anguera, M.T.; Pereira, A.; Araújo, D. Talent Identification and Development in Male Football: A Systematic Review. *Sport Med.* **2018**, *48*, 907–931. [CrossRef]
16. Larkin, P.; O'Connor, D. Talent identification and recruitment in youth soccer: Recruiter's perceptions of the key attributes for player recruitment. Sampaio J, editor. *PLoS ONE* **2017**, *12*, e0175716. [CrossRef]
17. Gonaus, C.; Müller, E. Using physiological data to predict future career progression in 14- to 17-year-old Austrian soccer academy players. *J. Sports Sci.* **2012**, *30*, 1673–1682. [CrossRef]
18. Pearson, D.T.; Naughton, G.A.; Torode, M. Predictability of physiological testing and the role of maturation in talent identification for adolescent team sports. *J. Sci. Med. Sport* **2006**, *9*, 277–287. [CrossRef]
19. Figueiredo, A.J.; Gonçalves, C.E.; Coelho, E.; Silva, M.J.; Malina, R.M. Youth soccer players, 11–14 years: Maturity, size, function, skill and goal orientation. *Ann. Hum. Biol.* **2009**, *36*, 60–73. [CrossRef] [PubMed]
20. Paul, D.J.; Nassis, G.P. Physical Fitness Testing in Youth Soccer: Issues and Considerations Regarding Reliability, Validity, and Sensitivity. *Pediatr. Exerc. Sci.* **2015**, *27*, 301–313. [CrossRef]
21. Fransen, J.; Bennett, K.J.M.; Woods, C.T.; French-Collier, N.; Deprez, D.; Vaeyens, R.; Lenoir, M. Modelling age-related changes in motor competence and physical fitness in high-level youth soccer players: Implications for talent identification and development. *Sci. Med. Footb.* **2017**, *1*, 203–208. [CrossRef]
22. Oancea, B. *Aspecte Practice ale Baschetului Scolar (Practical Aspects of School Basketball)*; Brasov, U.T., Ed.; Universitatea Transilvania Brasov: Brasov, Romania, 2016; pp. 15–25.
23. Hulse, M.; Morris, J.; Hawkins, R.; Hodson, A.; Nevill, A.; Nevill, M. A Field-Test Battery for Elite, Young Soccer Players. *Int. J. Sports Med.* **2012**, *34*, 302–311. [CrossRef] [PubMed]
24. Dugdale, J.H.; Arthur, C.A.; Sanders, D.; Hunter, A.M. Reliability and validity of field-based fitness tests in youth soccer players. *Eur. J. Sport Sci.* **2019**, *19*, 745–756. [CrossRef] [PubMed]
25. Buchheit, M. The 30-15 Intermittent Fitness Test: Accuracy for Individualizing Interval Training of Young Intermittent Sport Players. *J. Strength Cond. Res.* **2008**, *22*, 365–374. [CrossRef]
26. Sandford, G.N.; Laursen, P.B.; Buchheit, M. Anaerobic Speed/Power Reserve and Sport Performance: Scientific Basis, Current Applications and Future Directions. *Sport Med.* **2021**, *51*, 2017–2028. [CrossRef] [PubMed]
27. Slimani, M.; Nikolaidis, P.T. Anthropometric and physiological characteristics of male soccer players according to their competitive level, playing position and age group: A systematic review. *J. Sports Med. Phys. Fitness* **2019**, *59*, 141–163. [CrossRef] [PubMed]
28. Deprez, D.; Fransen, J.; Boone, J.; Lenoir, M.; Philippaerts, R.; Vaeyens, R. Characteristics of high-level youth soccer players: Variation by playing position. *J. Sports Sci.* **2015**, *33*, 243–254. [CrossRef]
29. Towlson, C.; Cobley, S.; Midgley, A.W.; Garret, A.; Parkin, G.; Lovell, R. Relative Age, Maturation and Physical Biases on Position Allocation in Elite-Youth Soccer. *Int. J. Sports Med.* **2017**, *38*, 201–209. [CrossRef] [PubMed]
30. Owoeye, O.B.; Akinbo, S.R.; Tella, B.A.; Olawale, O.A. Efficacy of the FIFA 11+ warm-up programme in male youth football: A cluster randomised controlled trial. *J. Sports Sci. Med.* **2014**, *13*, 321–328.
31. Durnin, J.V.G.A.; Womersley, J. Body fat assessed from total body density and its estimation from skinfold thickness: Measurements on 481 men and women aged from 16 to 72 Years. *Br. J. Nutr.* **1974**, *32*, 77–97. [CrossRef] [PubMed]
32. Zabaloy, S.; Freitas, T.T.; Carlos-Vivas, J.; Giráldez, J.C.; Loturco, I.; Pareja-Blanco, F.; Gálvez González, J.; Alcaraz, P.E. Estimation of maximum sprinting speed with timing gates: Greater accuracy of 5-m split times compared to 10-m splits. *Sport Biomech.* **2021**, 1–11. [CrossRef] [PubMed]
33. Rago, V.; Brito, J.; Figueiredo, P.; Ermidis, G.; Barreira, D.; Rebelo, A. The Arrowhead Agility Test: Reliability, Minimum Detectable Change, and Practical Applications in Soccer Players. *J. Strength Cond. Res.* **2020**, *34*, 483–494. [CrossRef] [PubMed]
34. Dos'Santos, T.; Thomas, C.; Jones, P.A.; Comfort, P. Assessing Asymmetries in Change of Direction Speed Performance: Application of Change of Direction Deficit. *J. Strength Cond. Res.* **2019**, *33*, 2953–2961. [CrossRef]
35. Sandford, G.N.; Kilding, A.E.; Ross, A.; Laursen, P.B. Maximal Sprint Speed and the Anaerobic Speed Reserve Domain: The Untapped Tools that Differentiate the World's Best Male 800 m Runners. *Sport Med.* **2019**, *49*, 843–852. [CrossRef] [PubMed]
36. Nikolaidis, P.T.; Vassilios Karydis, N. Physique and Body Composition in Soccer Players across Adolescence. *Asian J. Sports Med.* **2011**, *2*, 75. [CrossRef] [PubMed]
37. Malina, R.M.; Figueiredo, A.J.; Coelho-e-Silva, M.J. Body Size of Male Youth Soccer Players: 1978–2015. *Sport Med.* **2017**, *47*, 1983–1992. [CrossRef]

38. Gil, S.; Ruiz, F.; Irazusta, A.; Gil, J.; Irazusta, J. Selection of young soccer players in terms of anthropometric and physiological factors. *J. Sports Med. Phys. Fitness* **2007**, *47*, 25–32. [PubMed]
39. Leão, C.; Camões, M.; Clemente, F.M.; Nikolaidis, P.T.; Lima, R.; Bezerra, P.; Rosemann, T.; Knechtle, B. Anthropometric Profile of Soccer Players as a Determinant of Position Specificity and Methodological Issues of Body Composition Estimation. *Int. J. Environ. Res. Public Health.* **2019**, *16*, 2386. [CrossRef]
40. Rico-Sanz, J. Body Composition and Nutritional assessments in Soccer. *Int. J. Sport Nutr.* **1998**, *8*, 113–123. [CrossRef]
41. Gil, S.M.S.; Javier, G.; Ruiz, F.; Irazusta, A.; Irazusta, J. Physiological and anthropometric characteristics of young soccer players according to their playing position: Relevance for the selection process. *J. Strength Cond. Res.* **2007**, *21*, 438–445. [CrossRef]
42. Ziv, G.; Lidor, R. Physical Characteristics, Physiological Attributes, and On-Field Performances of Soccer Goalkeepers. *Int. J. Sports Physiol. Perform.* **2011**, *6*, 509–524. [CrossRef] [PubMed]
43. Mendez-Villanueva, A.; Buchheit, M.; Kuitunen, S.; Douglas, A.; Peltola, E.; Bourdon, P. Age-related differences in acceleration, maximum running speed, and repeated-sprint performance in young soccer players. *J. Sports Sci.* **2011**, *29*, 477–484. [CrossRef] [PubMed]
44. Al Haddad, H.; Simpson, B.M.; Buchheit, M.; Di Salvo, V.; Mendez-Villanueva, A. Peak Match Speed and Maximal Sprinting Speed in Young Soccer Players: Effect of Age and Playing Position. *Int. J. Sports Physiol. Perform.* **2015**, *10*, 888–896. [CrossRef]
45. Falk, B.; Bar-Or, O. Longitudinal Changes in Peak Aerobic and Anaerobic Mechanical Power of Circumpubertal Boys. *Pediatr. Exerc. Sci* **1993**, *5*, 318–331. [CrossRef]
46. Buchheit, M.; Samozino, P.; Glynn, J.A.; Michael, B.S.; Al Haddad, H.; Mendez-Villanueva, A.; Morin, J.B. Mechanical determinants of acceleration and maximal sprinting speed in highly trained young soccer players. *J. Sports Sci.* **2014**, *32*, 1906–1913. [CrossRef]
47. Loturco, I.; Bishop, C.; Freitas, T.T.; Pereira, L.A.; Jeffreys, I. Vertical Force Production in Soccer: Mechanical Aspects and Applied Training Strategies. *Strength Cond. J.* **2020**, *42*, 6–15. [CrossRef]
48. Loturco, I.; Nimphius, S.; Kobal, R.; Bottino, A.; Zanetti, V.; Pereira, L.A.; Jeffreys, I. Change-of direction deficit in elite young soccer players. *German J. Exercise and Sport Res.* **2018**, *48*, 228–234. [CrossRef]
49. Buchheit, M.; Mendez-Villanueva, A.; Simpson, B.M.; Bourdon, P.C. Match Running Performance and Fitness in Youth Soccer. *Int. J. Sports Med.* **2010**, *31*, 818–825. [CrossRef]
50. Haugen, T.; Tønnessen, E.; Hisdal, J.; Seiler, S. The role and development of sprinting speed in soccer. *Int. J. Sports physiol. Perform.* **2014**, *9*, 432–441. [CrossRef] [PubMed]
51. Mendez-Villanueva, A.; Buchheit, M.; Simpson, B.; Peltola, E.; Bourdon, P. Does on-field sprinting performance in young soccer players depend on how fast they can run or how fast they do run? *J. Strength Cond. Res.* **2011**, *25*, 2634–2638. [CrossRef]
52. Malina, R.M.; Bouchard, C.; Bar-Or, O. *Growth, Maturation, and Physical Activity*, 2nd ed.; Human Kinetics: Champaign, IL, USA, 2004.
53. Geithern, C.A.; Thomis, M.A.; Eynde, B.V.; Maes, H.H.; Loos, R.J.; Peeters, M.; Classens, A.L.M.; Vlietinck, R.; Malina, R.M.; Beunen, G.P. Growth in Peak Aerobic Power during Adolescence. *Med. Sci. Sport Exerc.* **2004**, *36*, 1616–1624.
54. Rowland, T.W. The "Trigger Hypothesis" for Aerobic Trainability: A 14-Year Follow-Up. Rowland TW, editor. *Pediatr. Exerc. Sci.* **1997**, *9*, 1–9. [CrossRef]
55. Harrison, C.B.; Gill, N.D.; Kinugasa, T.; Kilding, A.E. Development of Aerobic Fitness in Young Team Sport Athletes. *Sport Med.* **2015**, *45*, 969–983. [CrossRef]
56. Eriksson, B.O.; Gollnick, P.D.; Saltin, B. Muscle Metabolism and Enzyme Activities after Training in Boys 11–13 Years Old. *Acta Physiol. Scand.* **1973**, *87*, 485–497. [CrossRef]
57. Scott, B.R.; Hodson, J.A.; Govus, A.D.; Dascombe, B.J. The 30-15 Intermittent Fitness Test: Can It Predict Outcomes in Field Tests of Anaerobic Performance? *J. Strength Cond. Res.* **2017**, *31*, 2825–2831. [CrossRef]
58. Armstrong, N.; Welsman, J. Sex-Specific Longitudinal Modeling of Short-Term Power in 11- to 18-Year-Olds. *Med. Sci. Sport Exerc.* **2019**, *51*, 1055–1063. [CrossRef] [PubMed]
59. Armstrong, N.; Welsman, J. The Development of Aerobic and Anaerobic Fitness with Reference to Youth Athletes. *J. Sci. Sport Exerc.* **2020**, *2*, 275–286. [CrossRef]
60. Selmi, M.A.; Al-Haddabi, B.; Yahmed, M.H.; Sassi, R.H. Does Maturity Status Affect the Relationship Between Anaerobic Speed Reserve and Multiple Sprint Sets Performance in Young Soccer Players? *J. Strength Cond. Res.* **2020**, *34*, 3600–3606. [CrossRef] [PubMed]

International Journal of
Environmental Research
and Public Health

Article

Specific Physical Ability Prediction in Youth Basketball Players According to Playing Position

Jelena Ivanović [1,2], Filip Kukić [3], Gianpiero Greco [4,*], Nenad Koropanovski [5], Saša Jakovljević [6] and Milivoj Dopsaj [6,7]

1. Serbian Institute for Sport and Sports Medicine, 72 Kneza Višeslava Street, 11030 Belgrade, Serbia; jelena.ivanovic@rzsport.gov.rs
2. Faculty of Sport, University "Union—Nikola Tesla", Narodnih Heroja 30/I, 11070 Belgrade, Serbia
3. Police Sports Education Center, Abu Dhabi Police, Abu Dhabi 253, United Arab Emirates; filip.kukic@gmail.com
4. Department of Basic Medical Sciences, Neuroscience and Sense Organs, University of Study of Bari, 70121 Bari, Italy
5. Department of Criminalistics, University of Criminal Investigation and Police Studies, 11080 Belgrade, Serbia; nenad.koropanovski@kpu.edu.rs
6. Faculty for Sport and Physical Education, Belgrade University, 11000 Belgrade, Serbia; sasa.jakovljevic@fsfv.bg.ac.rs (S.J.); milivoj.dopsaj@gmail.com (M.D.)
7. Institute of Sport, Tourism and Service, South Ural State University, 454080 Chelyabinsk, Russia
* Correspondence: gianpierogreco.phd@yahoo.com

Abstract: This study investigated the hierarchical structure of physical characteristics in elite young (i.e., U17-U19) basketball players according to playing positions. In addition, their predictive value of physical characteristics was determined for the evaluation of players' physical preparedness. Sixty elite male basketball players performed 13 standardized specific field tests in order to assess the explosive power of lower limbs, speed, and change-of-direction speed. They were divided into three groups according to playing positions (guard [n = 28], forward [n = 22], center [n = 10]). The basic characteristics of the tested sample were: age = 17.36 ± 1.04 years, body height = 192.80 ± 4.49 cm, body mass = 79.83 ± 6.94 kg, and basketball experience = 9.38 ± 2.10 years for guards; age = 18.00 ± 1.00 years, body height = 201.48 ± 3.14 cm, body mass = 90.93 ± 9.85 kg, and basketball experience = 9.93 ± 2.28 years for forwards; and age = 17.60 ± 1.43 years; body height = 207.20 ± 3.29 cm, body mass = 104.00 ± 9.64 kg, and basketball experience = 9.20 ± 1.62 years for centers. For all playing positions factor analysis extracted three factors, which cumulatively explained 76.87, 88.12 and 87.63% of variance, respectively. The assessed performance measures were defined as significant ($p < 0.001$), with regression models of physical performance index (PP_{INDEX}). PP_{INDEX} of guards = −6.860 + (0.932 × t-test) − (1.656 × Acceleration 15 m) − (0.020 × Countermovement jump); PP_{INDEX} of forwards = −3.436 − (0.046 × Countermovement jump with arm swing) − (1.295 × Acceleration 15 m) + (0.582 × Control of dribbling); PP_{INDEX} of centers = −4.126 + (0.604 × Control of dribbling) − (1.315 × Acceleration 15 m) − (0.037 × Sargent jump). A model for the evaluation of physical performance of young basketball players has been defined. In addition, this model could be used as a reference model for selection procedures, as well as to monitor the efficacy of applied training programmes within the short, medium and long-term periodization.

Keywords: measurement; power test; speed test; change of direction speed test; guard; forward; center

1. Introduction

Body height, muscular power, speed, and strength are all important elements of the basketball player profile. Power, speed, and change of direction speed significantly contribute to the movement efficiency of basketball players with the ball and without it, as well as in technical and tactical elements of basketball game [1–3]. While body height is genetically predetermined, power, speed and change of direction speed are subject to training adaptation and could be used for the assessment of players' physical potential to overcome the challenges of a basketball game [3–5]. This is important in selection as well as training evaluation processes. Identification of younger players who have good physical potentials for basketball game reduces the probability of false selection, while early detection of deficits in the main physical abilities indicates that the training could be adjusted and may reduce the risk of unwanted injuries.

Managing the selection and training process depends on the adequacy of the assessment system in collecting information on athlete's or a team's training level in order to provide a precise evaluation of training level [6–8]. Furthermore, the usability of results obtained by the assessment depends on the specificity and sensitivity of the applied tests. The more specific the test is with regard to sport, the representation of competitive readiness is more valid [1,8,9]. If the correct data is collected from athletes, the coach can follow the trend in core physical abilities of basketball players through the age categories, and he can timely correct the training program to attain the short, medium, and long-term goals.

The available bibliography reveals the lack of design and use of specific tests to assess the physical attributes of the young basketball players, especially according to age categories and playing positions [1,8]. Growth and maturation affect physical abilities and physical performance [10–12], while different basketball positions present different demands and require specific physical attributes [13–15]. According to the results of a previous systematic review [1], the least common evaluated capacities in basketball players in literature are speed and agility. Tests of a generic nature have more frequently been used for assessing physical fitness in basketball players, e.g., aerobic and anaerobic capacity or jump performance [1,3,8,9,13–16]. Besides, only a few pieces of research have dealt with specific tests while dribbling the ball in basketball [1,8]. Consequently, talent identification, selection, and evaluation of training processes are very important parts of the systematic approach to the consistent competitive success of basketball team.

Considering the aforementioned factors, this study aimed to determine the hierarchical structure of physical characteristics in elite young (i.e., U17-U19) basketball players according to playing positions. In addition, their predictive value of physical characteristics was determined for the evaluation of players' physical preparedness. It was, firstly, hypothesized that significant hierarchical structure of physical abilities will be determined. Secondly, it was hypothesized that the highest ranked variables from the hierarchical structure could be the best predictors of players' physical performance.

2. Materials and Methods

2.1. Participants

The sample consisted of 60 male basketball players from the U19 and U17 Serbian national team. In order to obtain the most informative indicators to improve the technological process of managing, we recruited relatively large samples of participants to secure a sufficient statistical power. Besides, we selected a group of elite basketball players who won eight international medals in a period of four years during the biggest World and European competitions. They were allocated into three groups according to playing positions, as follows: Guards (n = 28, i.e., point guard and shooting guard), forwards (n = 22, i.e., small forward and power forward) and centers (n = 10). Basic characteristics of the tested sample were: age = 17.36 ± 1.04 years, 18.00 ± 1.00 years, 17.60 ± 1.43 years; body height = 192.80 ± 4.49 cm, 201.48 ± 3.14 cm, 207.20 ± 3.29 cm; body mass = 79.83 ± 6.94 kg, 90.93 ± 9.85 kg, 104.00 ± 9.64 kg; and training experience = 9.38 ± 2.10 years, 9.93 ± 2.28 years, 9.20 ± 1.62 years for guards, forwards and centers, respectively. All participants (athletes, coaches, and parents) were informed that their data may be used anonymously for scientific purposes and they were informed about the potential risks and discomforts associated with the investigation, and measurements were conducted out with their parental consent in line with the Helsinki Declaration. The Institutional Ethics Committee approved the research.

2.2. Measurement Procedure

All the tests were performed by the Serbian Institute of Sport and Sports Medicine at the beginning of the main pre-competitive mesocycle. Players were requested to refrain from strenuous exercise for at least 48 h, and from eating 2 h before testing. The testing session was carried out during morning hours between 10:00 and 12:00 a.m.

Before tests, players had performed a standardised warm-up, consisting of 5 min jogging, 5 min dynamic stretching, and 5 min of short acceleration-decelerations, gradual building of running velocity, submaximal jumping, and agility exercises. For the last five minutes of warm-up, players performed tests with submaximal intensity to potentiate specific muscles and joints. It is of note that the Serbian Institute of Sport and Sports Medicine asses the best Serbian athletes (i.e., members of the national teams) on a regular basis so the used tests were familiar to athletes. The assessment protocol for basketball athletes consists of sprint tests (with and without the ball), change of direction speed tests (with and without the ball), and vertical jump tests. Straight run speed, change of direction speed, and vertical jump heights were measured using Infrared timing gates and contact mat (Fusion sport, SmartJump and SmartSpeed, Grabba International Pty Ltd., Australia). The time of the run dribble was measured in seconds, with an accuracy of ±0.01 s. Jump tests are characterized by a very good test–retest reliability (in general Intraclass correlation coefficients are higher than 0.90) [13,16,17].

2.2.1. Sprint Tests

A 20 m sprint was performed from the standing position with the front foot placed on the line 30 cm behind the photocells. Times were recorded by infrared timing gates placed at the start, at 5 m (first-step quickness [Q5m]), 15 m (acceleration [A15m]), and finish line (Sprint 20 m [S20m]). Players performed the 20 m sprint two times without the ball and two times while dribbling the ball ($S20m_D$). The best time obtained from the trial was used for statistical analysis [8,13,18].

2.2.2. Change of Direction Speed with and without the Ball

The following five tests were used to assess change-of-direction speed: *t*-test (T_{TEST}), Slalom, Control dribble test (COND), Defensive movements test (DM), Change of direction speed test [2,3,8,16,18]. For the purpose of this study, we applied the standardized procedures used in the previous study [8].

T_{TEST} requires the athlete to move in a T-shaped pattern. According to earlier described procedures [8,13,16,18], the photocells were placed at the starting line and in line with central cone positioned 9 m away from starting position. The athletes started from the standing position, and ran forward 9 m as fast as possible. Then, they shuffled 4.5 m laterally to the left without crossing their feet to another cone. After touching this cone, they shuffled laterally 9 m to the right to a third cone, touched it, side shuffled back to the middle cone, and ran backward to where they started.

In case of Slalom (Slalom), and Slalom while dribbling the ball ($Slalom_D$), each participant started the test with his feet behind the baseline of the basketball court. Subjects were required to run (dribble), as fast as possible up and down the course around the three cones placed linearly with 2.6 m distance. They performed two trials with and without the ball and the fasters ones were used for the analysis [8].

The COND test was performed at the 5.8 m × 3.6 m rectangle polygon marked by six cones positioned as follows: two at both ends of the free-throw lane, two at the baseline aligned with those at the free-throw line, one in the middle of the rectangle, and one that marked the starting point [8]. The athletes were required to navigate dribbling through a course as fast as possible. The athletes started with their non-dominant hand on the non-dominant side of cone A. They dribbled with non-dominant hand to the non-dominant side of cone B, and then proceed to cone C and cone D, dribbling with the dominant hand. The course continued with the non-dominant hand to cone E and then with the dominant hand to cone F where the test was completed (Figure 1). Three trials were completed for the test. The first was a practice trial and the sum of the second (starting with non-dominant hand) and third trials (starting with dominant hand) was retained for analysis.

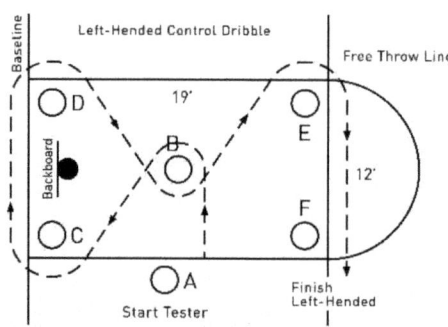

Figure 1. Schematic illustration of the Control of dribbling test. A, B, C, D, E, F—cones; dotted arrow—direction of dribbling.

The DM was used to evaluate the performance of defensive movements. It was performed at the same rectangle polygon as COND, but two cons were positioned at the halfway point of the longer edges of the rectangle. This test was carried following the procedure described in a previous study [8]. The player was required to shuffle laterally without crossing the feet in a sequence of seven changes of direction. Whenever the players changed direction, they were required to touch the floor and execute a drop-step (changing direction by moving the trailing foot in the sliding motion to the new direction (Figure 2). The fastest of the two trials was recorded for the analysis.

A change of direction test (COD) consists of a sprint with several changes of direction. The athletes started in the triple-threat position behind the baseline of the basketball court. Players were required to run (dribble) and to change direction as fast as possible to two different lines, namely, the near free-throw line (5.8 m) and the half-court line (14 m). The athletes sprinted to the free-throw line first and back to the baseline, then to the half-court line and back to the baseline, and finally to the free-throw line again and back to the baseline. Before every change of direction, they were required to step on the line with one foot. After changing direction, they were required to change the dribbling hand. Each athlete was allowed two trials with and without the ball and the fastest one was retained for analysis. Two players performed the test at the same time to encourage maximal effort [8].

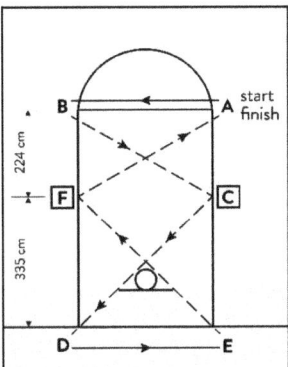

Figure 2. Schematic illustration of the Defensive movements test. A, B, C, D, E, F—cones; dotted arrow—direction of movements.

2.2.3. Vertical Jumps

The following four types of vertical jump were performed: Sargent jump (SGJ), Squat Jump (SJ), Countermovement jump with arm swing (CMJ_{AS}) and Countermovement jump (CMJ). In case of SGJ, the athlete chalked the end of his/her fingertips, stood sideways onto the wall, kept both feet on the ground, reached up as high as possible with one hand and marked the wall with the tips of the fingers (M1). From a static position, they jumped as high as possible and marked the wall with the chalk on their fingers (M2). The distance between M1 and M2 was used to calculate jump height. The athlete repeated the test 2 times [2]. SJ and CMJ vertical jump height were performed according to well-established procedures [13,16–18]. In short, SJ was performed from the 90-degree semi-squat position using only the maximal contraction of lower limbs, while CMJ was performed utilizing the energy from the stretch–shortening cycle. In SJ and CMJ, hands were kept at the hips for the entire movement to eliminate any influence of the arm. A CMJ_{AS} was performed the same way as CMJ but players were allowed to swing with their hands upward. Two maximal jumps were performed, and the highest result was registered as the final result.

2.3. Statistical Procedures

The mean and standard deviation values for each test were calculated for each subgroup (guards, forwards, and centers). For all the tests involving several trials, test–retest reliability was assessed using intraclass correlation coefficients (ICC). For defining the structure, i.e., real qualitative relationships between variables, the principal component analysis (PCA) was used. A multivariate assessment of the adequacy of the raw data was carried out using the Kaiser-Meyer-Olkin (KMO) measure of sampling adequacy and Bartlett's Tests of sphericity ($p < 0.001$), for which statistical significance was expressed in terms of a chi-square (χ^2). Eigenvalues > 1 were considered for the extraction of principal components. A Direct Oblimin rotation method was performed in order to identify the high correlation of components and guarantee that each principal component offered different information [19]. A criterion variable from factor analysis was used as a representation of the player's multidimensional physical performance index (PP_{INDEX}) according to playing position so each player could be compared against the criterion value for their playing position [20]. Multiple regression analysis with the PP_{INDEX} as the criterion variable and the performance test variables as predictor variables determined the unique evaluation of specific preparedness of basketball players according to playing position [20]. Statistical significance for all analyses was defined as $p < 0.001$. All statistical operations were carried out by applying the Microsoft® Office Excel 2010 and the SPSS for Windows, Release 20.0 (Copyright © SPSS Inc., Chicago, IL, USA, 1989–2002).

3. Results

Results for the descriptive statistics (Mean and Standard deviation) of the observed characteristics with regard to different playing position and Intraclass correlation coefficients (ICCs) for relative test–retest reliability are shown in Table 1. It can be observed that, in terms of positions, forwards were faster than guards and centers in Q5m and Q5m$_D$, while guards were faster than forwards and centers in the majority of change-of-direction speed and sprint tests. In addition, guards achieved a greater jump height compared with forwards and centers. The average inter-item correlation in all variables described mutual correlation within a correlation matrix at a statistically significant level at $p < 0.001$ (Bartlett's test of Sphericity) and ranged between 0.689 for A15m$_D$ and 0.992 for CMJ, indicating a good reliability.

Table 1. Descriptive statistics and Intraclass correlation coefficients.

	Guard	Forward	Center	Test–Retest Reliability	
	Mean ± SD	Mean ± SD	Mean ± SD	Average Int-Item Correlation	Bartlett's Test of Sphericity
Q5m (s)	1.817 ± 0.413	1.606 ± 0.522	1.820 ± 0.547	0.977	F = 42.775 *
Q5m$_D$ (s)	1.883 ± 0.426	1.721 ± 0.647	1.905 ± 0.587	0.732	F = 3.735 *
A15m (s)	1.185 ± 0.378	1.445 ± 0.520	1.372 ± 0.489	0.814	F = 5.384 *
A15m$_D$ (s)	1.212 ± 0.396	1.494 ± 0.573	1.437 ± 0.501	0.689	F = 3.218 *
S20m (s)	3.002 ± 0.117	3.052 ± 0.180	3.194 ± 0.128	0.967	F = 30.166 *
S20m$_D$ (s)	3.096 ± 0.154	3.215 ± 0.292	3.344 ± 0.162	0.866	F = 7.488 *
T$_{TEST}$ (s)	10.321 ± 0.402	10.481 ± 0.711	11.282 ± 0.695	0.970	F = 33.330 *
DM (s)	18.038 ± 0.860	18.351 ± 1.252	19.601 ± 1.377	0.960	F = 25.079 *
Slalom (s)	4.117 ± 0.178	4.199 ± 0.253	4.443 ± 0.213	0.956	F = 22.797 *
Slalom$_D$ (s)	4.214 ± 0.180	4.349 ± 0.272	4.629 ± 0.292	0.959	F = 24.441 *
COD (s)	11.922 ± 0.463	12.114 ± 0.787	12.582 ± 0.905	0.927	F = 13.773 *
COD$_D$ (s)	12.482 ± 0.404	12.713 ± 0.825	13.036 ± 0.653	0.953	F = 21.394 *
COND(s)	12.852 ± 0.840	13.144 ± 1.144	13.643 ± 1.180	/	/
CMJ (cm)	41.16 ± 6.20	39.15 ± 5.93	35.79 ± 4.33	0.992	F = 119.140 *
CMJ$_{AS}$ (cm)	48.77 ± 6.30	47.62 ± 6.76	43.67 ± 5.60	0.984	F = 63.837 *
SJ (cm)	34.59 ± 5.77	33.49 ± 5.70	30.28 ± 4.69	0.974	F = 38.620 *
SGJ (cm)	49.34 ± 6.61	48.05 ± 7.66	43.02 ± 3.72	0.929	F = 14.044 *

* T$_{TEST}$: t test total time; DM: Defensive movements; S20m$_D$: Sprint with dribbling 20 m; COD$_D$: Change of direction with dribbling; Slalom: Slalom; Slalom$_D$: Slalom with dribbling; A15m$_D$: Acceleration with dribbling 15 m; COD: Change of direction; COND: Control of dribbling; S20m: Sprint 20 m; A15m: Acceleration 15 m; Q5m$_D$: Quickness with dribbling 5 m; Q5m: Quickness 5 m; CMJ: Countermovement jump without arm swing; SJ: Squat jump; CMJ$_{AS}$: Countermovement jump with arm swing; SGJ: Sargent jump; * p values: $p = 0.000$.

The KMO showed a high statistical significance of multivariate adequacy of the given variables at the level of 0.561 ($\chi^2 = 848.338$, $p < 0.001$) for guards, at the level of 0.677 ($\chi^2 = 689.135$, $p = 0.001$) for forwards, and at the level of 0.558 ($\chi^2 = 744.770$, $p = 0.001$). For all playing positions, the factor analysis extracted three significant factors (Table 2), which cumulatively explained 76.867, 88.123 and 87.633% of variance in guards, forwards, and centers, respectively.

Table 2. Saturated factors with the structure indicators of the explained variance.

Factor	Extraction Sums of Squared Loadings								
	Total			% of Variance			Cumulative %		
	Guard	Forward	Center	Guard	Forward	Center	Guard	Forward	Center
1	6.719	9.997	11.333	39.523	58.804	66.664	39.523	58.804	66.664
2	3.644	3.899	2.465	21.435	22.936	14.499	60.958	81.739	81.162
3	2.705	1.085	1.100	15.909	6.384	6.471	76.867	88.123	87.633

Table 3 shows the structure matrix with the variable saturation for each playing position. Measured physical characteristics provide a similar factor structure for each position, with a lateral change of direction speed being highly ranked in guards, jumping ability in forwards, and change of direction speed between baseline and free-throw line in centers. The second factor included straight-run speed measures with and without the ball for all three positions. The third factor included a jumping performance in guards, change of direction speed while dribbling the ball, defensive movement in forwards, and jumping performance in centers (with emphasis on jumps with arm swings). This suggests that the measured characteristics with regard to different playing positions have different structures in the function of isolated factors, which may be attributed to their adaptation to specific training process.

Table 3. Factor analysis structure matrix for each playing position.

Factor	Guard		Forward		Center	
	Variables	Value	Variables	Value	Variables	Value
1st factor	T_{TEST}	0.804	CMJ_{AS}	−0.966	COND	0.962
	DM	0.783	CMJ	−0.957	COD_D	0.940
	$S20m_D$	0.762	S20	0.934	COD	0.916
	Slalom	0.759	T_{TEST}	0.918	Slalom	0.891
	$Slalom_D$	0.754	SJ	−0.912	T_{TEST}	0.887
	COD	0.749	SGJ	−0.897	$Slalom_D$	0.848
	COD_D	0.749	Slalom	0.878	DM	0.834
	COND	0.720	$Slalom_D$	0.834	S20m	0.821
	S20m	0.624	COD_D	0.823	$S20m_D$	0.818
2nd factor	A15m	−0.984	A15m	−0.983	A15m	0.993
	$Q5m_D$	0.984	$A15m_D$	−0.977	$A15m_D$	0.990
	Q5m	0.980	Q5m	0.967	Q5m	−0.980
	$A15m_D$	−0.973	$Q5m_D$	0.959	$Q5m_D$	−0.969
3rd factor	CMJ	0.974	COND	0.869	SGJ	0.949
	CMJ_{AS}	0.944	DM	0.846	CMJ_{AS}	0.943
	SJ	0.886	COD	0.828	CMJ	0.871
	SGJ	0.813	$S20m_D$	0.827	SJ	0.860

T_{TEST}: t-test total time; DM: Defensive movements; $S20m_D$: Sprint with dribbling 20 m; COD_D: Change of direction with dribbling; Slalom: Slalom; $Slalom_D$: Slalom with dribbling; $A15m_D$: Acceleration with dribbling 15 m; COD: Change of direction; COND: Control of dribbling; S20m: Sprint 20 m; A15m: Acceleration 15 m; $Q5m_D$: Quickness with dribbling 5 m; Q5m: Quickness 5 m; CMJ: Countermovement jump without arm swing; SJ: Squat jump; CMJ_{AS}: Countermovement jump with arm swing; SGJ: Sargent jump.

The results of the defined regression analysis have shown high predictive potential for PP_{INDEX} of guards (AdjR^2 = 0.893, F = 165.597, p < 0.001, Standard Error of the Estimate = 0.33), forwards (AdjR^2 = 0.896, F = 170.577, p < 0.001, Standard Error of the Estimate = 0.31), and centers (AdjR^2 = 0.875, F = 138.412, p < 0.001, Standard Error of the Estimate = 0.34). The final mathematical models for evaluation of PP_{INDEX} of guards, forwards, and centers is as follows:

PP_{INDEX} of guards = −6.860 + (0.932 × T test) − (1.656 × Acceleration 15 m) − (0.020 × Countermovement jump),

PP_{INDEX} of forwards = −3.436 − (0.046 × Countermovement jump with arm swing) − (1.295 × Acceleration 15 m) + (0.582 × Control of dribbling),

PP_{INDEX} of centers = −4.126 + (0.604 × Control of dribbling) − (1.315 × Acceleration 15 m) − (0.037 × Sargent jump).

In this manner, by a very simple mathematical model, coaches could be provided with a tool for the evaluation of players' physical preparedness according to position, in terms of a deterministic, fully controlled system.

The regression analysis further reduced the multidimensionality of players' physical preparedness to the most essential components that predict the PP_{INDEX} of young players with high precision. The best predictors in guards included T_{TEST}, A15m, CMJ. The best predictors in forwards were CMJ_{AS}, A15m, COND. The best predictors in centers were COND, A15m, and SGJ. Thus, the highest-ranked variables in each factor were the best predictors of PP_{INDEX} for the corresponding positions. The regression model allows for the qualitative and quantitative evaluation of players on the three investigated positions (See Figure 3).

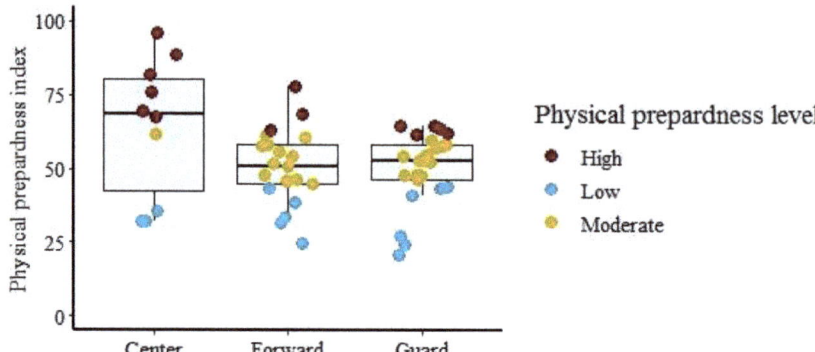

Figure 3. Positioning of players according to playing position from the aspect of specific preparation level.

4. Discussion

This study investigated the hierarchical structure of physical characteristics in elite young basketball players and evaluated their predictive value in the evaluation of players' physical preparedness. The main findings showed that specific change of direction speed performance was the highest-ranked characteristic in guards, specific jumping performance was the highest-ranked characteristic in forwards, while the control of specific movements while dribbling the ball was the highest-ranked characteristic in centers. Moreover, a significant prediction model for the evaluation of physical preparedness was defined for each playing position. These findings are of high importance as they provide a screening tool for selection and training evaluation processes.

Considering the structure of the basketball game, players are required to perform numerous technical–tactical elements characterized by agile movements in space in a planned manner or as a response to the opponent's actions [21]. Shooting guards within their roles and duties perform a higher number of lateral shuffles, forward and backward sprints on relatively bigger area than centers or small forwards. This could be attributed to the role in the game that guards have, such as losing the defender further from the basket by quick directional changes with and without the ball and quick return to defend the basket. Therefore, running speed, agility, and rapid recovery are critical fitness components, particularly for this position [9,13–15].

Forwards, on the other hand, typically perform a high number of jumps whether offensively to score the basket or defensively when rebounding, which is also emphasized in the training process. Thereby, jumping characteristics are of high importance for this position. Basketball players typically perform 40–50 jumps per game, generating force rapidly to perform various tasks such as rebounding, blocking opponent shot attempts, and creating elevation for a jump shot [2]. The movement structure of CMJ and CMJ_{AS} corresponds to the bilateral vertical jumps that players most often perform when they are shooting from the distance to advance their ball release height and when they are trying to block the opponent. In addition, forwards are also responsible for the quick return to defence and to defend the space by quick lateral shuffles.

Centers are usually referred to as "frontcourt", often acting as their team's primary below-the-basket rebounders and shot blockers. They also receive passes to take inside shots for which they must control their body, opponent, and the ball. Therefore, it is not surprising that centers, as major players on the team, require a high level of control of the specific movement with the ball to maintain their body position when battling with the opponents for important positions under the basket. However, considering the game rules that do not allow staying below the basket longer than 5 s, center is required to move constantly in a square-shaped space from the baseline to the free-throw line. They need to be agile compared to other centers so they could position themselves in a good position repeatedly.

The second factor consisting of acceleration and sprint for all positions indicated the importance of these characteristics for basketball players. Short sprints represent a multidimensional movement skill that requires an explosive concentric and SSC force production of a number of lower-limb muscles [22]. During a game, the players are rarely in a situation where they have to sprint across the whole court. Therefore, sprint tests over shorter distances and acceleration are more appropriate to administer to basketball players [3,8,22]. Indeed, to a large degree (certainly more than power and agility) speed is genetically predetermined, thereby fast players are selected rather than "made fast", especially considering the sample of this study that consisted of elite players for their age category [23]. This does not reduce the importance of this factor, but additionally suggests that the applied strength and conditioning training could include strength and power exercises that may additionally improve running speed and acceleration or reduce the risk of injury caused by these activities [24–26]. It is interesting to mention that center were slightly faster than forwards in the A15 and A15$_D$ tests (Table 1). However, if an index of technical efficiency is calculated (the ratio between the A15 and A15$_D$ tests), it may be concluded that forwards are still more efficient than centers. Although there are no data in the available literature on the 15 m acceleration test in basketball, results of some previous research showed no significant difference between playing position in the 20 m sprint [9,13]. Even more, these authors suggested that despite their size and weight, centers are as fast as smaller players. Besides that, significant effect of playing position on sprint performance increase in shorter (10 m and shorter) and longer (20 m and longer) distance [13,14] which strongly support our findings.

The last factor is vertical jump performances in guards and centers, showing that these characteristics, although not dominant, are a very important pillar of a basketball player's physical preparedness. The most representative variable in the third factor was the countermovement jump for guards and Sargent jump for centers. The obtained differences in hierarchy of this factor correspond to differences in how guards and centers perform jumps in the game. Guards are typically jumping free from the opposing player (i.e., no contact with opposing player) and from previously performed movement, while centers are typically jumping from the spot, while in contact with the opposing player with one hand and reaching high with the other to block, rebound or score. Unlike guards and centers, the third factor extracted change of direction speed and speed variables, whereby most representatives were the control of dribbling. This is not surprising, given that forwards often perform dribble penetration to advance to the basket [9,13–15].

There is a scarcity of studies that address the specific characteristics of physical fitness in basketball players, even though the battery of basic performance tests are widely used. The reason for that could lie in a fact that possibility of providing a sample of the best selected players for the age category is low. Research dealing with the hierarchical structure and equation of specification in relation to specific performance tests in basketball is practically non-existent in the available literature. The lack of reference to these problems has certainly reduced the possibility to compare our findings with other studies. Data on the defined latent structure of standard indicators of situational efficiency in the game of basketball [27] or in relation to the tests of generic nature [28] can be found in the available literature. The results of that research have shown that the highest total variance in 13 male and 13 female semiprofessional basketball players was represented by aerobic capacity and in-game physical conditioning [28]. In addition, as one of the main limitations of this study, the authors mentioned the need for the inclusion of specific basketball-field tests (e.g., agility with and without the ball, anaerobic capacity) to evaluate the physical performance of basketball players [28]. In relation to the research that used similar methodology [20], the results suggest that it is possible to create sport- position-specific prediction model for evaluation physical preparedness.

Limitations

However, some limitations should be acknowledged when interpreting the results of this research. An apparent limitation of this study is the results may not be generalized to other age groups or females. In order to apply the obtained results in general, it is necessary to conduct extensive research that includes the examination of physical ability on a large sample of basketball players, of different ages, competitive level and for both genders. Another limitation originates from the cross-sectional design that does not allow for the identification of the effects of physical activity from the initial selection of the subjects.

5. Conclusions

The results obtained in this research show that the measured characteristics with regard to different playing positions have different structures in the function of isolated factors under the influence of different mechanisms with regard to the training process. As a factor analysis has a primarily discriminatory character, the first factor with observed variables where the basketball players differ most is the most important one. Specific change direction agility abilities, i.e., specific locomotion on the court is the most important element within guard position in elite youth basketball players. Specific jumping ability is the most important element within the forward position. Control of specific movement with the ball is the most important element within center position.

Practical Applications

With the multiple regression analysis, the influence of the selected variables on the physical performance index (PP_{INDEX}) was obtained, and the equation of specific basketball preparedness according to playing position. This index represents the position of the participant on a hypothetical scale with a minimum of 0 and a maximum of 100 points. In this manner, it is possible to obtain relevant data in relation to physical ability characteristics and, indirectly, to obtain the performance potential of a given athlete. Thus, a useful means for the level of physical fitness determination of youth basketball players has been obtained, as well as a comprehensive reference model for use in selection procedures, screening candidates, or to monitor the efficacy of training regimes.

Author Contributions: Conceptualization, J.I. and M.D.; methodology, J.I., M.D. and S.J.; validation, F.K. and G.G.; formal analysis, J.I., M.D. and F.K.; investigation, J.I. and S.J.; resources, J.I., G.G., F.K. and S.J.; data curation, J.I., G.G., F.K. and N.K.; writing—original draft preparation, J.I., M.D., G.G. and F.K.; writing—review and editing, J.I., F.K., G.G. and N.K.; supervision, M.D., F.K. and G.G.; project administration, J.I. and F.K. All authors have read and agreed to the published version of the manuscript.

Funding: This research received no external funding.

Institutional Review Board Statement: The study was conducted according to the guidelines of the Declaration of Helsinki and approved by the Ethics Commission of the Faculty of Sport and Physical Education, University of Belgrade (protocol code 482-2, February 2011).

Informed Consent Statement: Informed consent was obtained from all subjects involved in the study.

Data Availability Statement: The data presented in this study are available on request from the corresponding author.

Acknowledgments: The paper was realized as part of project III47015 sponsored by Ministry of Science and Technological Development in the Republic of Serbia.

Conflicts of Interest: The authors declare no conflict of interest.

References

1. Mancha-Triguero, D.; García-Rubio, J.; Calleja-González, J.; Ibáñez, S.J. Physical fitness in basketball players: A systematic review. *J. Sports Med. Phys. Fit.* **2019**, *59*, 1513–1525. [CrossRef]
2. Wen, N.; Dalbo, V.J.; Burgos, B.; Pyne, D.B.; Scanlan, A.T. Power testing in basketball: Current practice and future recommendations. *J. Strength Cond. Res.* **2018**, *32*, 2686–2700. [CrossRef]
3. Zarić, I.; Dopsaj, M.; Marković, M. Match performance in young female basketball players: Relationship with laboratory and field tests. *Int. J. Perform. Anal. Sport* **2018**, *18*, 90–103. [CrossRef]
4. Stojanović, E.; Stojiljković, N.; Scanlan, A.T.; Dalbo, V.J.; Berkelmans, D.M.; Milanović, Z. The activity demands and physiological responses encountered during basketball match-play: A systematic review. *Sports Med.* **2018**, *48*, 111–135. [CrossRef] [PubMed]
5. Ferioli, D.; Rampinini, E.; Bosio, A.; La Torre, A.; Azzolini, M.; Coutts, A.J. The physical profile of adult male basketball players: Differences between competitive levels and playing positions. *J. Sports Sci.* **2018**, *36*, 2567–2574. [CrossRef] [PubMed]
6. Belyakova, A.; Gorskaya, I. Psychomotor abilities as a factor of future success in athletes. *Hum. Sports Med.* **2021**, *21*, 102–107. [CrossRef]
7. Zatsiorsky, V.M.; Kraemer, W.J. *Science and Practice of Strength Training*, 2nd ed.; Human Kinetics: Champaign, IL, USA, 2006.
8. Ivanović, J.; Dopsaj, M.; Jakovljević, S.; Karalejić, M. Relationship between isometric neuromuscular function of the leg extensors with performance tests in basketball. *Russ. Open Med. J.* **2019**, *8*, 1–8. [CrossRef]
9. Drinkwater, E.J.; Pyne, D.B.; McKenna, M.J. Design and interpretation of anthropometric and fitness testing of basketball players. *Sports Med.* **2008**, *38*, 565–578. [CrossRef] [PubMed]
10. Toselli, S.; Campa, F.; Maietta Latessa, P.; Greco, G.; Loi, A.; Grigoletto, A.; Zaccagni, L. Differences in Maturity and Anthropometric and Morphological Characteristics among Young Male Basketball and Soccer Players and Non-Players. *Int. J. Environ. Res. Public Health* **2021**, *18*, 3902. [CrossRef]
11. Towlson, C.; Cobley, S.; Parkin, G.; Lovell, R. When does the influence of maturation on anthropometric and physical fitness characteristics increase and subside? *Scand. J. Med. Sci. Sports* **2018**, *28*, 1946–1955. [CrossRef] [PubMed]
12. Arede, J.; Fernandes, J.; Moran, J.; Norris, J.; Leite, N. Maturity timing and performance in a youth national basketball team: Do early-maturing players dominate? *Int. J. Sports Sci. Coach* **2021**, *16*, 722–730. [CrossRef]
13. Delextrat, A.; Cohen, D. Strength, power, speed, and agility of women basketball players according to playing position. *J. Strength Cond. Res.* **2009**, *23*, 1974–1981. [CrossRef]
14. Köklü, Y.; Alemdaroğlu, U.; Koçak, F.; Erol, A.; Findikoğlu, G. Comparison of Chosen Physical Fitness Characteristics of Turkish Professional Basketball Players by Division and Playing Position. *J. Hum. Kinet.* **2011**, *30*, 99–106. [CrossRef]
15. Boone, J.; Bourgois, J. Morphological and Physiological Profile of Elite Basketball Players in Belgium. *Int. J. Sports Physiol. Peform.* **2013**, *8*, 630–638. [CrossRef] [PubMed]
16. Jakovljević, S.; Karalejić, M.; Brini, S.; Ben Abderrahman, A.; Boullosa, D.; Hackney, A.C.; Zagatto, A.M.; Castagna, C.; Bouassida, A.; Granacher, U.; et al. Effects of a 12-Week Change-of-Direction Sprints Training Program on Selected Physical and Physiological Parameters in Professional Basketball Male Players. *Int. J. Environ. Res. Public Health* **2020**, *17*, 8214. [CrossRef]
17. Markovic, G.; Dizdar, D.; Jukic, I.; Cardinale, M. Reliability and factorial validity of squat and countermovement jump tests. *J. Strength Cond. Res.* **2004**, *18*, 551–555. [CrossRef]
18. Maggioni, M.A.; Bonato, M.; Stahn, A.; La Torre, A.; Agnello, L.; Vernillo, G.; Castagna, C.; Merati, G. Effects of Ball Drills and Repeated-Sprint-Ability Training in Basketball Players. *Int. J. Sports Physiol. Perform.* **2019**, *14*, 757–764. [CrossRef]
19. Rojas-Valverde, D.; Pino-Ortega, J.; Gómez-Carmona, C.D.; Rico-González, M. A Systematic Review of Methods and Criteria Standard Proposal for the Use of Principal Component Analysis in Team's Sports Science. *Int. J. Environ. Res. Public Health* **2020**, *17*, 8712. [CrossRef]
20. Majstorović, N.; Dopsaj, M.; Grbić, V.; Savić, Z.; Vićentijević, A.; Aničić, Z.; Zadražnik, M.; Toskić, L.; Nešić, G. Isometric Strength in Volleyball Players of Different Age: A Multidimensional Model. *Appl. Sci.* **2020**, *10*, 4107. [CrossRef]
21. Abdelkrim, N.B.; Chaouachi, A.; Chamari, K.; Chtara, M.; Castagna, C. Positional role and competitive-level differences in elite-level men's basketball players. *J. Strength Cond. Res.* **2010**, *24*, 1346–1355. [CrossRef] [PubMed]
22. Markovic, G.; Mikulic, P. Neuro-Musculoskeletal and Performance Adaptations to Lower Extremity Plyometric Training. *Sports Med.* **2010**, *4*, 859–895. [CrossRef]
23. Ben-Zaken, S.; Eliakim, A.; Nemet, D.; Meckel, Y. Genetic Variability Among Power Athletes: The Stronger vs. the Faster. *J. Strength Cond. Res.* **2019**, *33*, 1505–1511. [CrossRef] [PubMed]
24. Young, W.B. Transfer of strength and power training to sports performance. *Int. J. Sports Physiol. Perform.* **2006**, *1*, 74–83. [CrossRef] [PubMed]
25. Zouita, S.; Zouita, A.B.M.; Kebsi, W.; Dupont, G.; Ben Abderrahman, A.; Ben Salah, F.Z.; Zouhal, H. Strength training reduces injury rate in elite young soccer players during one season. *J. Strength Cond. Res.* **2016**, *30*, 1295–1307. [CrossRef]
26. Case, M.J.; Knudson, D.V.; Downey, D.L. Barbell squat relative strength as an identifier for lower extremity injury in collegiate athletes. *J. Strength Cond. Res.* **2020**, *34*, 1249–1253. [CrossRef] [PubMed]
27. Sporiš, G.; Šango, J.; Vučetić, V.; Mašina, T. The latent structure of standard game efficiency indicators in basketball. *Int. J. Perform. Anal. Sport* **2006**, *6*, 120–129. [CrossRef]
28. Gómez-Carmona, C.D.; Mancha-Triguero, D.; Pino-Ortega, J.; Ibáñez, S.J. Exploring Physical Fitness Profile of Male and Female Semiprofessional Basketball Players through Principal Component Analysis—A Case Study. *J. Funct. Morphol. Kinesiol.* **2021**, *6*, 67. [CrossRef] [PubMed]

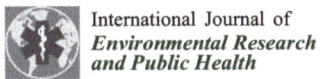

Article

The Influence of Cultural Experiences on the Associations between Socio-Economic Status and Motor Performance as Well as Body Fat Percentage of Grade One Learners in Cape Town, South Africa

Eileen Africa [1], Odelia Van Stryp [1] and Martin Musálek [2],*

[1] Faculty of Medicine and Health Sciences, Stellenbosch University, Private Bag X1, Matieland 7602, South Africa; africa@sun.ac.za (E.A.); odeliavs@sun.ac.za (O.V.S.)
[2] Faculty of Physical Education and Sport, Charles University, José Martího 31 Praha 6, 162 52 Veleslavín, Czech Republic
* Correspondence: musalek@ftvs.cuni.cz

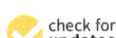

Citation: Africa, E.; Stryp, O.V.; Musálek, M. The Influence of Cultural Experiences on the Associations between Socio-Economic Status and Motor Performance as Well as Body Fat Percentage of Grade One Learners in Cape Town, South Africa. *Int. J. Environ. Res. Public Health* **2022**, *19*, 121. https://doi.org/10.3390/ijerph19010121

Academic Editors: Francesco Campa and Gianpiero Greco

Received: 30 November 2021
Accepted: 17 December 2021
Published: 23 December 2021

Publisher's Note: MDPI stays neutral with regard to jurisdictional claims in published maps and institutional affiliations.

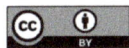

Copyright: © 2021 by the authors. Licensee MDPI, Basel, Switzerland. This article is an open access article distributed under the terms and conditions of the Creative Commons Attribution (CC BY) license (https://creativecommons.org/licenses/by/4.0/).

Abstract: Fundamental movement skills (FMS), physical fitness (PF) and body fat percentage (BF%) are significantly related to socio-economic status (SES). However, it remains unclear why previous studies have had different findings regarding the direction of the association between SES and FMS, PF and BF%. A suggested explanation is that the direction of the link can be influenced by cultural experiences and traditions. Therefore, the aim of the current study was to investigate links between SES and FMS, PF, BF% of Grade One learners from two different ethno-geographic areas in Cape Town, South Africa. Grade One children (n = 191) (n = 106 boys and n = 85 girls; age (6.7 ± 0.33)) from different socio-economic areas in Cape Town, South Africa, were selected to participate in the study. South African schools are classified into five different quintiles (1 = poorest and 5 = least poor public schools). For this study, two schools were selected, one from quintile 2 and the other from quintile 5. BF% was assessed according to Slaughter's equation. FMS were measured using the Gross Motor Development Test-2 (TGMD-2) and PF via five tests: 1. dynamic strength of lower limb (broad jump); 2. dynamic strength of upper limb and trunk (throwing a tennis ball); 3. speed agility (4 × 10 m shuttle running); 4. cardiorespiratory fitness (20 m shuttle run endurance test (Leger test)) and 5. flexibility (sit and reach test). An analysis of covariance (ANCOVA) found that BF% and WHtR were significantly greater in children with higher SES (Z = 6.04 p < 0.001; Hedg = 0.54), (Z = 3.89 p < 0.001; Hedg = 0.32). Children with lower SES achieved significantly better TGMD-2 standard scores in the locomotor subtest, compared to their peers with higher SES. In the object control subtest, no significant SES-related difference was found. However, ANCOVA showed that girls performed better in FMS than boys. In PF, the main effect of SES was observed in dynamic strength of trunk and upper limb (throwing) and flexibility, where children with lower SES performed significantly better. No significant difference was found in cardiorespiratory performance (CRP) (Beep test), even though children with lower SES achieved better results. Results from the current study suggest that links between SES, PF, FMS and body fat percentage in children seem to be dependent on cultural and traditional experiences. These experiences should therefore be included as an important factor for the development of programmes and interventions to enhance children's lifelong motor behaviour and health strategies.

Keywords: fundamental movement skills; physical fitness; adiposity; children; cultural experiences; socio-economic status

1. Introduction

The development of fundamental movement skills (FMS) and health-related physical fitness (PF) during childhood presents important health parameters [1] for promoting long-term positive and sustainable health trajectories, especially in obesity prevention [2].

In addition, a large body of studies have verified that children with lower PF or FMS, regardless of geographic specification, tend to be overweight or obese [3–7], even at preschool age [8,9]. The aforementioned health trajectories are expounded in the Stodden model [10], which explains that reciprocal relations between motor competence, FMS, health-related physical fitness, self-perceiving of motor competences and physical activity play a key role. However, the Stodden model does not consider the socioeconomic status (SES) of individuals, although SES has been found to be an important indicator in the prevalence of obesity as well as in PF and FMS development [11].

Previous research that focused on the relationship between obesity and SES in school-age children has not brought clear results. While studies that include children from North America, Australia and Europe suggest that lower SES is significantly associated with a risk of overweightness and obesity [9,12,13], other studies from Brazil or Korea did not find any such relationship [14,15]. Moreover, research done in South America [16], the Arab world [17], and particularly in Africa [11,18,19] showed reversed patterns. It means that children with high SES displayed a higher chance of being overweight and obese. One of the suggested explanations for this research disconformity is that obesity is strongly associated with globalization, i.e., expansion of economic and social interdependence [19,20], which is generally not the same in different world regions.

When we look at the association between motor performance and SES, one of the basic assumptions is that children with lower SES tend to have motor developmental delays [21–23]. However, as noted in previous paragraph, the association between SES and particularly FMS levels seems to be culturally dependent. While in well-developed or Western countries a positive association between SES and FMS was found from pre-school age [24–26], in developing or middle developed countries, including South African (SA) children, the results are not clear [27], since those with lower SES usually performed better in FMS than their peers with higher SES [28]. In addition, Armstrong [29] concluded that in SA children an inverse relation between SES and FMS was observed only for kicking the ball, which is a specific variable performed within the manipulation construct. Moreover, it is important to realize that FMS development is evidently sex-dependent during pre-school and school age. Girls usually have better locomotor skills, while boys perform better in object control [24,30,31], regardless of income status of country [32]. Pienaar et al. [5] found the same pattern in SA first grade children recruited from households with low-to-middle SES. Interestingly, some studies on pre-school [33] and school children [34] found that FMS level is rather associated with SES in girls; however, when considering age, the relation is reversed.

PF as physical readiness showed itself to be also sex-dependent when, regardless of SES, boys outperformed girls in the majority of PF capacity tests (strength, endurance, speed) from preschool age, while girls achieved better results in flexibility [35–37]. However, results from studies investigating the association between PF and SES are inconsistent and copy the trends of results found in the association between SES and FMS. While the majority of previous results suggest that children with higher SES tend to perform better in PF compared to peers with lower SES [29,38,39], some studies did not find any significant association [40]. Moreover, [41] or Freitas et al. [42], for instance, showed that children with higher SES performed better in speed and strength but significantly worse in flexibility and endurance compared to children from lower SES schools.

Previous findings have indicated that the currently accepted relationships between obesity, FMS and PF, for example within the Stodden model, can be strongly influenced by SES, but not always in the same direction and not similarly in both sexes. If we consider obesity prevalence, FMS and PF level from preschool age to be significantly inversely related to the amount and intensity of physical activity [43,44], then sociocultural factors, as suggested by [45], such as the opportunities for leisure time physical activities, personal family support or physical transportation habits [46], might explain why SES is differently associated with motor development or obesity prevalence in school children in culturally different countries. Therefore, the researchers deemed it essential to highlight the importance of SES in the interpretation of the links between motor development and the prevalence of obesity in children. This information might fundamentally contribute to adequate long-term motor and overall development of children.

The aim of the current study was therefore to investigate the differences in FMS, PF and body fat percentage (BF%) between Grade One learners from different ethno-geographic backgrounds in Cape Town, South Africa.

2. Materials and Methods

2.1. Participants

The measurements took place in the first term of the school year. Two Grade One classes from schools in Cape Town, South Africa, were selected to participate in the study. The two schools were based in different socio-economic areas and categorized under different quintiles. All South African schools are classified in five different quintiles based on financial resources (Table 1).

Table 1. Background to South African quintile system.

Quintile	Description
1–3	No fees schools
4–5	Fee paying schools

Quintile 1 schools are the poorest, while quintile 5 schools are the least poor [47]. In the current study, school B is categorized under quintile 5 and school W quintile 2. Prior to the data collection, ethical approval was obtained from the Research Ethics committee (#8456) and the study was conducted according to the guidelines of the Declaration of Helsinki. Permission was sought from the Education Department to approach the schools. Written consent from the parents/guardians and assent from the children were obtained for participation in the study. A total of $n = 191$ ($n = 106$ boys and $n = 85$ girls; 6.1 ± 0.4 years old) Grade One children participated in the study.

According to Table 2, all age categories were normally distributed. As reported by the two-way ANOVA, children from school "W" were significantly younger than children from school "B" ($F_{137\ 1} = 8.71$ $p = 0.004$; $\eta^2 \rho = 0.07$). The results also showed no significant difference between girls and boys.

Table 2. Descriptive Age—School "W"—lower SES and School "B"—higher SES.

School	Boys Mean	Girls Mean
School "W" lower SES	6.6 ± 0.3	6.54 ± 0.33
School "B" higher SES	6.75 ± 0.39	6.73 ± 0.29

Data are presented as mean ± SD.

2.2. Instruments

a. Anthropometric measurements:

All anthropometry parameters were measured by one trained examiner using the Eston and Reilly [48] manual. Body height was measured using a portable anthropometer P375 (Co. TRYSTOM, spol. s r.o./1993–2015 www.trystom.cz, accessed on 23 November 2021), with measurements taken to the nearest 0.1 cm. Body weight was measured using a medical calibrated scale TPLZ1T46CLNDBI300, with body weight recorded to the nearest 0.1 kg. Skinfolds were done using subscapular and triceps with the Harpenden skinfold caliper, with an accuracy of 0.2 mm. Waist circumference was measured with metal measuring tape with an accuracy of 0.1 cm.

Body fat percentage was estimated according to [49]'s equations. Previous studies showed that Slaughter's equation is adequate alternative used in children for estimating percentage of body fat where Dual-energy X-ray absorptiometry (DXA) is not available [50–54].

The following equations were used [49]:

For white males with a sum of skinfolds less than 35 mm the following equation was used:

$$BF\% = 1.21 \times (tric + subsc) - 0.008 \times (tric + subsc)^2 - 1.7$$

For black males with a sum of skinfolds less than 35 mm the following equation was used:

$$BF\% = 1.21 \times (tric + subsc) - 0.008 \times (tric + subsc)^2 - 3.2$$

For all females with a sum of skinfolds less than 35 mm the following equation was used:

$$BF\% = 1.33 \times (tric + subsc) - 0.013 \times (tric + subsc)^2 - 2.5$$

For males with a sum of skinfolds higher than 35 mm the following equation was used:

$$BF\% = 0.783 \times (tric + subsc) + 1.6$$

For females with a sum of skinfolds higher than 35 mm the following equation was used:

$$BF\% = 0.546 \times (tric + subsc) + 9.7$$

Note: tric: triceps skinfold; subsc: subscapular skinfold

The waist-to-height ratio index was used as an indirect parameter for estimating abdominal fat. Several studies have indicated that WHtR is useful in clinical and population health as it identifies children with excessive body fat [55] and greater risk of developing weight-related cardiovascular disease at an early age [56]. The waist circumference was measured at the midway between the lowest border of the rib cage and the upper iliac crest to the nearest 0.1 cm [57]. Anthropometric measurements were conducted before lunch time.

b. Fundamental movement skills:

Fundamental movement skills were evaluated with the Test for Gross Motor Development-2 (TGMD-2) [58], which is a valid and reliable measurement of FMS [59–64]. The TGMD-2 assesses proficiency in two motor-area composites (Table 3):

Table 3. TGMD-2 composites.

Locomotor	Object Control
Run	Striking a stationary ball
Hop	Stationary dribble
Horizontal jump	Catch
Leap	Overhand throw
Gallop	Kick
Slide	Underhand roll

Inter-rater reliability for the TGMD-2 was ensured by two experienced *Kinderkineticists; both received the same videos of 10 children and had to score them according to the TGMD-2 criteria and manual.

The testing took place in the specific school's hall. A clear demonstration of every skill was given by the assistant at the station. Children had one practice trial and two formal test trials. The formal testing trials were video recorded (consent was given) in order to properly score each participant afterwards according to the criteria of the TGMD-2 manual. The raw scores were converted to standard scores considering the sex and age of participants. Each child received a number for all the measurements and the number was shown on the video.

*Kinderkinetics is a profession that aims to develop and enhance the total well-being of children between 0–12 years of age, by stimulating, rectifying and promoting age-specific motor and physical development [65].

After the testing, the videos were transferred from the tablets to a memory stick and analysed on a computer by the researcher and assistants.

c. Physical fitness:

Physical fitness was measured using five widely accepted tests [66–68], namely broad jump for dynamic strength of lower limbs; throwing a tennis ball for dynamic strength of upper limb and trunk; 4 × 10 m shuttle running for speed agility; 20 m shuttle run endurance test (Leger test) for cardiorespiratory fitness; and a sit and reach test for flexibility. The examiners explained and demonstrated all PF tests to the children before the tests commenced. Detailed descriptions of the PF tests used are available at: (https://ftvs.cuni.cz/FTVS-726-version1-physical_fitness_tests_description.pdf, accessed on 23 November 2021).

2.3. Statistical Analysis

Normality of data was analysed using the Shapiro–Wilk test as well as coefficients of skewness and kurtosis. Variance–covariance homogeneity was verified using the Box M test, and the regression slopes homogeneity via the significance of between-subjects effects [69]. To accommodate age differences between children with different SES, an analysis of covariance 2 (SES) × 2 (sex) using age as covariate was applied. ANCOVA was used for selected variables, which passed all assumptions for its application (height, weight, skeletal robustness and physical fitness tests).

The effect size was estimated by the partial eta squared ($\eta^2 p$) with range <0.05 small effect size; 0.06–0.25 moderate effect size; 0.26–0.50 large effect size; >0.50 very large effect size [70,71] and Hedge's g range <0.2 small effect size; 0.21–0.50 moderate effect size; 0.51–0.80 large effect size; >0.80 very large effect size. All data was analysed in NCSS2007 [72].

3. Results

3.1. Anthropometry

Since age is significantly correlated with personal height, the current study used analysis of covariance (ANCOVA) (r = 0.47), where age was determined as a covariate. Although children with lower SES were significantly younger, the difference in height in relation to SES between children with lower SES and higher SES remained significant. It means that even though the age of participants was significantly related to height ($F_{137\,1}$ = 25.63 $p < 0.001$; $\eta^2 p$ = 0.20), children with lower SES were still significantly shorter compared to their peers with higher SES ($F_{137\,1}$ = 40.23 $p < 0.001$; $\eta^2 p$ = 0.30). Furthermore, weight was poorly correlated with age; therefore, a simple two-way ANOVA was performed, which showed that children with lower SES were significantly lighter ($F_{137\,1}$ = 39.74 $p < 0.001$; $\eta^2 p$ = 0.30). No significant differences were found for height and weight between boys and girls. Body fat percentage and WHtR were not normally distributed (Table 4. BF% was found to be significantly greater in children with higher SES (Z = 6.04 $p < 0.001$; Hedg = 0.54). In addition, girls had a greater BF% compared to boys (Z = 4.41 $p < 0.001$; Hedg = 0.38). The same differences were found in WHtR, where children with higher SES had significantly greater values (Z = 3.89 $p < 0.001$; Hedg = 0.32). In contrast to BF%, no significant differences were found between boys and girls.

Table 4. Descriptive height and weight frame indices.

Variables	SES			
	Boys (Lower SES)	Boys (Higher SES)	Girls (Lower SES)	Girls (Higher SES)
Height cm	116.6 ± 4.13 *** (a)	122 ± 3.98	115.3 ± 5.97 *** (b)	122 ± 5.37
Weight kg	20.4 ± 3.3 *** (a)	24.2 ± 3.12	19.7 ± 2.8 *** (b)	26.1 ± 7.7
BF%	10.6 ± 3.8 *** (a)	16.4 ± 4.9	14.6 ± 3.4 *** (b)	20.9 ± 8.1
WHtR	0.43 ± 0.03 *** (a)	0.45 ± 0.03	0.44 ± 0.03 *** (b)	0.47 ± 0.05

Data are presented as mean ± SD, *** $p < 0.001$. (a) Significant difference between boys with lower and boys with higher SES. (b) Significant difference between girls with lower and girls with higher SES.

3.2. Fundamental Movement Skills

In general, children with lower SES achieved significantly better TGMD-2 standard scores compared to their peers with higher SES ($F_{137\ 1} = 6.73$ $p = 0.01$; $\eta^2\rho = 0.05$). Detailed analysis, however, revealed the effect of SES only in the locomotor subtest, where children with lower SES achieved significantly better scores ($F_{137\ 1} = 6.11$ $p = 0.014$; $\eta^2\rho = 0.05$). In the object control subtest, no significant difference was found between children with higher and lower SES; however, ANCOVA showed that girls performed better than boys ($F_{137\ 1} = 20.78$ $p < 0.001$; $\eta^2\rho = 0.16$) (Table 5).

Table 5. TGMD-2 performance considering SES and sex of children.

TGMD Skills	Boys (Lower SES)	Boys (Higher SES)	Girls (Lower SES)	Girls (Higher SES)
Object control	10.2 ± 1.5	10.1 ± 2.1	11.8 ± 2.2 *** (b)	11.6 ± 2.0 ***
Locomotor	10.1 ± 3.0 * (a)	8.3 ± 1.8	9.6 ± 2.2 * (b)	8.8 ± 2.3
Overall TGMD-2	20.3 ± 3.0 ** (a)	18.4 ± 3.2	21.4 ± 3.0 ** (b)	20.4 ± 3.2

Data are presented as mean ± SD * $p < 0.05$ ** $p < 0.01$ *** $p < 0.001$. (a) Significant difference between boys with lower and boys with higher SES. (b) Significant difference between girls with lower and girls with higher SES.

3.3. Physical Fitness

Not all results from the physical fitness tests were significantly related to SES. The effect of SES on muscular strength of trunk and upper limb—throwing (right) ($F_{137\ 1} = 24.64$ $p < 0.001$; $\eta^2\rho = 0.18$), throwing (left) ($F_{137\ 1} = 4.68$ $p = 0.03$; $\eta^2\rho = 0.04$) and flexibility ($F_{137\ 1} = 12.37$ $p < 0.001$; $\eta^2\rho = 0.09$)—was found mainly in children with lower SES. In dynamic strength of lower limbs (broad jump) and agility (shuttle run—4 × 10 m), sex was found to have an effect, but not SES. In both tests, girls achieved lower dynamic strength of lower limbs ($F_{137\ 1} = 10.04$ $p = 0.002$; $\eta^2\rho = 0.08$) and were significantly slower compared to boys ($F_{137\ 1} = 8.16$ $p = 0.005$; $\eta^2\rho = 0.06$). No significant difference was found in cardiorespiratory performance (CRP) (Beep test), even though children with lower SES achieved better results (Table 6).

Table 6. Physical fitness performance considering SES and sex of children.

	SES			
	Boys		Girls	
	(Lower SES)	(Higher SES)	(Lower SES)	(Higher SES)
Broad jump (cm)	113.0 ± 16 ** (c)	120.6 ± 17.3 ** (c)	105.2 ± 20.2	108.0 ± 19.9
Shuttle run—4 × 10 m (s)	13.8 ± 1.1 ** (c)	13.7 ± 1.3 ** (c)	14.3 ± 0.8	14.4 ± 1.3
Throw right (m)	15.1 ± 5.5 *** (a)	10.7 ± 3.7	10.0 ± 4.0 *** (b)	7.6 ± 1.6
Throw left (m)	7.2 ± 3.0	6.5 ± 2.4	6.7 ± 2.8	5.9 ± 1.5
Beep test (No. of tracks)	16.8 ± 9.6	15.2 ± 6.9	15.8 ± 6.7	13.6 ± 6.7
Flexibility (cm)	19.5 ± 4.7 ***	15.6 ± 4.9	20.7 ± 5.0 ***	18.4 ± 5.9

Data are presented as mean ± SD ** $p < 0.01$ *** $p < 0.001$. (a): Significant difference between boys with lower and boys with higher SES. (b): Significant difference between girls with lower and girls with higher SES. (c) Significant difference considering sex regardless of SES.

4. Discussion

The aim of the current study was to investigate the differences in FMS, PF and BF% between Grade One learners from different socio-economic backgrounds in Cape Town, South Africa. After controlling for differences in sex and age, SES was positively associated with height and weight.

Children with higher SES had significantly higher BF% and were heavier. Similar results brought [73] to the conclusion that overweight and obese children in China are from a higher SES. Possible reasons include available amounts of food, less physical activity and a more sedentary lifestyle in children with higher SES. These findings are contrary to the results of [74,75], who found that weight and body mass index in relation to obesity of British children with lower SES were higher compared to their peers with higher SES. In addition, higher weight and body fat are considered as a sign of wealth in certain countries [76,77]. For instance, children with high SES in Sub-Saharan Africa also displayed a higher chance of being overweight and obese [78]. These findings contradict previous studies [9,12,13] which found an inverse association between SES and body fat. A multiethnic study [79] found that obese African black girls had the highest self-esteem compared to Asian or European peers. Specifically, overweight South African black women perceive themselves as more attractive [80,81]. A very recent qualitative study [82] revealed in South African adult participants that fatness is connected with symbols of prosperity and beauty rather than with health problems. A different view of body status is also known from other cultures such as China, where being too thin is the same problem as being too fat [83]. This suggests that socio-cultural environments including ethnicity or race can link SES to weight gain and obesity status differently, as proposed by [84].

4.1. Fundamental Movement Skills

The results of this study indicate that children with lower SES performed significantly better than their higher-SES peers according to the standard scores of total TGMD-2 and the locomotor subtest of the TGMD-2, but not in the object control subtest. This finding is in contrast with most previous research from the Western world, where children with higher SES outperformed their lower-SES counterparts in FMS [85,86]. For instance, [34], who performed their study in Australia, and [86], who performed theirs in the United States, suggested that the differences could be attributed to lower cardiorespiratory fitness, physical activity levels, absence of weekly physical education, fewer opportunities for perceptual motor experiences and disadvantaged communities that lack facilities. Nevertheless, our study found no significant difference in CRF in relation to SES (see in detail below PF part). Furthermore, our findings are consistent with a recent South African study by [87], which was carried out in a very similar demographic environment and which also stated that rural low-income children had significantly better TGMD-2 standard scores. This negates the notion that children with lower SES naturally perform worse in overall FMS than children with higher SES due to limited access to safe outdoor playing and equipment [88] or safe places to be active in the community or to sporting equipment at home [89]. A possible reason for this finding is that children with lower SES often engage in unstructured moderate-to-vigorous physical activity with limited teacher facilitation compared to their higher-SES peers, and this might positively influence the development of FMS [87,90,91]. Children with lower SES in South Africa also tend to spend a greater amount of time in active transportation to and from schools [92,93]. Therefore, according to some authors, different findings in terms of FMS levels in South Africa compared to western, educated, industrialized, rich and democratic (WEIRD) countries can be attributed to South Africa's unique socio-cultural environment [94,95].

4.2. Physical Fitness

In the physical fitness measurement, only the performances in upper limb throwing and flexibility were significantly inversely associated with SES, where children with lower SES achieved significantly better results. These findings support those of [96], who suggested that the relationship between PF and SES has not been consistently clarified.

Some studies, however, did observe a significant positive link between SES and aspects of PF (muscle strength, aerobic fitness, muscular endurance and speed) [97–99]. In contrast, [99] did not find any provable associations between SES and PF, and other studies [39,100] even found that children with lower SES outperformed their peers with higher SES in flexibility and endurance. The results of the current study are more consistent with the conclusions of the latter.

Inverse associations between SES and throwing could be explained by differences in opportunities and content of physical activity [29]. It has been known for more than 70 years that the way children with different SES spend their leisure time depends on their SES environment [101–103]. Children with higher SES usually spend leisure time participating in organized commercial physical activities [104], while children with lower SES tend to play simple group games with cheap equipment in the street [105,106]. In addition, this spontaneous type of PA usually has implicit motor learning characteristics [107], where a high number of repetitions of motor activity without explicit instructions is considered typical. Implicit motor learning for acquiring motor skills such as overhead throwing has been shown to significantly influence automation and accuracy of the movement pattern [108–110]. Therefore, the range of the movement experience and the defined motor pattern, along with how this motor pattern (overhead throwing) was acquired in low SES children, could explain the inverse association between SES and performance in throwing a tennis ball found in the current study. This assumption would also support previous suggestions that children with lower SES seem to have better coordination [97,111–113]. On the other hand, the results of the current study do not support the South African study conducted by [29], who did not find any significant differences in the throwing of a cricket ball in 6–7-year-old children when taking SES into consideration. That study included more than 600 children from five provinces in that age category. Since the participants of the current study were only from one province, sample variability could be a reason for the discrepancy in the results.

In the flexibility measurement, children with lower SES showed better results. These are in line with the findings of [29,39]. This difference could be explained by genetic differences in collagen alleles associated with physical performance/functional tests [114], even though relationships between genotypes and clinical phenotypes are not well defined. Chan et al. [115] found that in African Americans, collagen development COL1A1 COL1A2 responsible for development of bone, cartilage and tendons seemed to be evolutionarily different from European Americans, increasing flexibility in the African American population.

If one looks at differences in performance of each component of PF, it is evident in the research that children with higher SES are stronger and have better muscular explosiveness [97,111] which is in line with the current study's findings.

Results from the cardiorespiratory fitness (CRF) test showed that children with lower SES performed better in the multistage fitness test. However, due to the large variability of results in each category of children (higher SES, lower SES, boys and girls), the differences were not significant. Nevertheless, studies from Sub-Saharan Africa found better CRF in children with lower SES compared to their higher-SES counterparts [42,105,116]. The better CRF of children with lower SES could be explained by their daily habits and physical activity profile compared to children with higher SES. Prista et al. [117] found that increased physical activity of children with lower SES was mainly due to higher demands of daily physical activities, such as walking, running and playing. VandenDriessche et al. [96] and Micklesfield et al. [103] found that children with lower SES walked to school and engaged in more physical activity on the way to and from school. On the other hand, these children spend less time in moderate-to-vigorous physical activity at school and in clubs [105]. Furthermore, Micklesfield et al. [103] suggested that children with lower SES spend more active time at the household and community level, which implies less sedentary behaviour in this social environment. These findings seem to be dependent on the social and cultural environment because the result of better PF in children with lower SES is contrary to results from studies done in the Western world, where children with lower SES performed repeatedly worse in CRF tests [99,112].

In summary, our findings should be used for the development of further education strategies with the aim of preventing obesity and properly controlling child's motor development and physical fitness, which are influenced by SES differently considering specifics of socio-cultural and ethno-graphic experiences. It means, for instance, the extension of PE classes at least in primary school education, along with changes in content or implementation of active breaks or socialization games. This seems, according to [118], to be positively influenced by the conjunction of school and family environments intervention programs.

4.3. Strength and Limitations

To the best of our knowledge, this is the first study of its kind to consider traditional and cultural experiences (including ethnographic differences) as an important factor influencing the direction of the links between SES, motor performance and body fat percentage in children. An additional strength of this study is that the sample (two different socio-economic/ethno-graphic groups) was specifically defined and selected according to the guidelines (www.education.gov.za, accessed on 16 December 2021) stipulated by the Department of Basic Education in South Africa. However, the research sample was selected from a narrow population in the Western Cape; therefore, the results of this study may not be completely representative of all Grade One children in the Western Cape. Furthermore, the absence of biological maturation status of the children in this study might be a limitation because previous studies have suggested that biological maturation influences performance in strength and endurance [119,120]. However, most previous studies did not consider this parameter in similar age samples. In the current study children with higher SES were significantly taller and heavier, which suggests that they might be advanced in their biological maturation. Unfortunately, there is no valid and reliable method in South Africa to assess biological maturation for this age group in multi-ethnic populations. We suggest that future research explore the inclusion of biological maturation when assessing motor performance and BF% in children with different SES.

5. Conclusions

In contrast to Western countries, children with lower SES in the current study were leaner, had lower BF% and performed significantly better in FMS (specifically in their locomotor skills) compared to their higher SES peers. Furthermore, children with lower SES performed significantly better in dynamic strength of the trunk and upper limb and flexibility compared to children with higher SES. Therefore, we suggest that links between SES, PF, FMS and BF% in children seem to be dependent on country-specific cultural and ethno-graphic experiences. The uniqueness of cultural experiences with regard to SES should be included as an important factor for the development of programmes and interventions to enhance lifelong motor behaviour and health strategies for children.

Author Contributions: Conceptualization, O.V.S., E.A. and M.M.; data curation, O.V.S. and M.M.; investigation, O.V.S. and M.M.; methodology, M.M.; project administration, E.A.; writing—original draft, O.V.S., E.A. and M.M. All authors have read and agreed to the published version of the manuscript.

Funding: This study was endorsed by the project PROGRES Q19, Social-Sciences Aspects of Human Movement Studies II and financially supported by the institutions involved.

Institutional Review Board Statement: The study was conducted according to the guidelines of the Declaration of Helsinki, and approved by the Research Ethics Committee (Humanities) of Stellenbosch University # 8456, 22 February 2019.

Informed Consent Statement: Written informed consent was obtained from all subjects involved in the study.

Data Availability Statement: The data set is available at https://www.researchgate.net/publications/create?publicationType=dataset, accessed on 17 December 2021.

Conflicts of Interest: The authors declare no conflict of interest.

References

1. Robinson, L.E.; Stodden, D.F.; Barnett, L.M.; Lopes, V.P.; Logan, S.W.; Rodrigues, L.P.; D'Hondt, E. Motor competence and its Effect on Positive Development Trajectories of Health. *Sports Med.* **2015**, *45*, 1273–1284. [CrossRef]
2. Cattuzzo, M.T.; Henrique, R.; Re, A.H.N.; De Oliveira, I.S.; Melo, B.M.; De Sousa Moura, M.; De Araujo, R.C.; Stodden, D. Motor competence and health related physical fitness in youth: A systematic review. *J. Sci. Med. Sport* **2016**, *19*, 123–129. [CrossRef]
3. Lubans, D.R.; Morgan, P.J.; Cliff, D.P.; Barnett, L.M.; Okely, A.D. Fundamental Movement Skills in Children and Adolescents. *Sports Med.* **2010**, *40*, 1019–1035. [CrossRef]
4. Vameghi, R.; Shams, A.; Dehkordi, P.S. The effect of age, sex and obesity on fundamental motor skills among 4 to 6 years-old children. *Pak. J. Med. Sci.* **2013**, *29*, 586–589. [CrossRef]
5. Pienaar, A.E.; Van Reenen, I.; Weber, A.M. Sex differences in fundamental movement skills of a selected group of 6-year-old South African children. *Early Child Dev. Care* **2016**, *186*, 1994–2008. [CrossRef]
6. Niederer, I.; Kriemler, S.; Zahner, L.; Bürgi, F.; Ebenegger, V.; Marques-Vidal, P.; Puder, J.J. BMI Group-Related Differences in Physical Fitness and Physical Activity in Preschool-Age Children. *Res. Q. Exerc. Sport* **2012**, *83*, 12–19. [CrossRef] [PubMed]
7. Abdelkarim, O.; Ammar, A.; Trabelsi, K.; Cthourou, H.; Jekauc, D.; Irandoust, K.; Hoekelmann, A. Prevalence of underweight and overweight and its association with physical fitness in Egyptian schoolchildren. *Int. J. Environ. Res. Public Health* **2020**, *17*, 75. [CrossRef]
8. Musalek, M.; Kokstejn, J.; Papez, P.; Scheffler, C.; Mumm, R.; Czernitzki, A.; Koziel, S. Impact of normal weight obesity on fundamental motor skills in pre-school children aged 3 to 6 years. *J. Biol. Clin. Anthropol.* **2017**, *74*, 203–212. [CrossRef] [PubMed]
9. Ogden, C.L.; Carroll, M.D.; Curtin, L.R.; Lamb, M.M.; Flegal, K.M. Prevalance of High Body Mass Index in US children and Adolescents, 2007–2008. *J. Am. Med. Assoc.* **2010**, *303*, 242–249. [CrossRef] [PubMed]
10. Stodden, D.F.; Goodway, J.D.; Langendorfer, S.J.; Roberton, M.; Rudisill, M.E.; Garcia, C.; Garcia, L.E.A. Developmental Perspective on the Role of Motor Skill Competence in Physical Activity: An Emergent Relationship. *J. Mot. Competence Phys. Act.* **2008**, *60*, 290–306. [CrossRef]
11. Choukem, S.; Kamdeu-Chedeu, J.; Leary, S.D.; Mboue-Djieka, Y.; Nebongo, D.N.; Akazong, C.; Mapoure, Y.N.; Hamilton-Shield, J.P.; Gautier, J.; Mbanya, J.C. Overweight and obesity in children aged 3–13 years in urban Cameroon: A cros-sectional study of prevalence and association with socio-economic status. *BMC Obes.* **2017**, *4*, 1–8. [CrossRef] [PubMed]
12. Rao, D.P.; Kropac, E.; Do, M.T.; Roberts, K.C.; Jayaraman, G.C. Childhood overweight and obesity trends in Canada. *Health Promot. Chronic Dis. Prev. Can. Res. Policy Pract.* **2016**, *36*, 194. [CrossRef] [PubMed]
13. Hardy, L.; Mihrshahi, S.; Gale, J.; Drayton, B.A.; Bauman, A.; Mitchell, J. 30-year trends in overweight, obesity and waist-to-height ratio by socioeconomic status in Australian children, 1985 to 2015. *Int. J. Obes.* **2017**, *41*, 76–82. [CrossRef] [PubMed]
14. Matsudo, V.K.R.; Ferrari, G.L.D.M.; Araújo, T.L.; Oliveira, L.C.; Mire, E.; Barreira, T.V.; Katzmarzyk, P. Socioeconomic status indicators, physical activity, and overweight/obesity in Brazilian children. *Rev. Paul. De Pediatr.* **2016**, *34*, 162–170. [CrossRef]
15. Lee, H.J.; Kim, S.H.; Choi, S.H.; Lee, J.S. The association between socioeconomic status and obesity in Korean children: An analysis of the Fifth Korea National Health and Nutrition Examination Survey (2010–2012). *Pediatric Gastroenterol. Hepatol. Nutr.* **2017**, *20*, 186–193. [CrossRef]
16. Herrera, J.C.; Lira, M.; Kain, J. Socioeconomic vulnerability and obesity in Chilean schoolchildren attending first grade: Comparison between 2009 and 2013. *Rev. Chil. Pediatr.* **2017**, *88*, 736–743. [CrossRef]
17. Al-Hussaini, A.; Bashir, M.S.; Khormi, M.; AlTuraiki, M.; Alkhamis, W.; Alrajhi, M.; Halal, T. Overweight and obesity among Saudi children and adolescents: Where do we stand today? *Saudi J. Gastroenterol.* **2019**, *25*, 229–235. [CrossRef] [PubMed]
18. Griffiths, P.L.; Rousham, E.K.; A Norris, S.; Pettifor, J.M.; Cameron, N. Socio-economic status and body composition outcomes in urban South African children. *Arch. Dis. Child.* **2008**, *93*, 862–867. [CrossRef]

19. Ljungvall, Å. *The Freer the Fatter? A Panel Study of the Relationship between Body-Mass Index and Economic Freedom*; Lund University: Lund, Switzerland, 2013.
20. Costa-Font, J.; Mas, N. Globesity? The effects of globalization on obesity and caloric intake. *Food Policy* **2016**, *64*, 121–132. [CrossRef]
21. Bobbio, T.G.; Morcillo, A.M.; Filho, A.D.B.; Goncalves, V.M.G. Factors Associated with Inadequate Fine Motor Skills in Brazilian Students of Different Socioeconomic Status. *Percept. Mot. Skills* **2007**, *105*, 1187–1195. [CrossRef]
22. Handal, J.A.; Lozoff, B.; Breilh, J.; Harlow, D.S. Effect of community of residence on neurobehavioral development in infants and young children in a flower-growing region of Ecuador. *Environ. Health Perspect.* **2007**, *115*, 128–133. [CrossRef]
23. Grantham-McGregor, S.M.; Fernald, L.C.; Kagawa, R.M.C.; Walker, S. Effects of integrated child development and nutrition interventions on child development and nutritional status. *Ann. N. Y. Acad. Sci.* **2014**, *1308*, 11–32. [CrossRef]
24. Hardy, L.; King, L.; Farrell, L.; Macniven, R.; Howlett, S. Fundamental movement skills among Australian preschool children. *J. Sci. Med. Sport* **2010**, *13*, 503–508. [CrossRef] [PubMed]
25. Pienaar, A.E.; Visagie, M.; Leonard, A. Proficiency at Object Control Skills by Nine- to Ten-Year-Old Children in South Africa: The NW-Child Study. *Percept. Mot. Ski.* **2015**, *121*, 309–332. [CrossRef] [PubMed]
26. Mülazimoglu-Ballo, Ö. Motor Proficiency and Body Mass Index of Preschool Children: In Relation to Socioeconomic Status. *J. Educ. Train. Stud.* **2017**, *4*, 237–243.
27. Aalizadeh, B.; Mohamadzadeh, H.; Hosseini, F.S. Fundamental movement skills among Iranian primary school children. *J. Fam. Reprod. Health* **2014**, *8*, 155–159.
28. Venter, A.; Pienaar, A.E.; Coetzee, D. Extent and nature of motor difficulties based on age, ethnicity, gender and socio-economic status in a selected group of three-to five-year-old children. *S. Afr. J. Res. Sport Phys. Educ. Recreat.* **2015**, *37*, 169–183.
29. Armstrong, M.E.G.; Lambert, E.V.; Lambert, M.I. Physical fitness of South African primary school children, 6 to 13 years of age: Discovery vitality health of the Nation study. *Percept. Mot. Skills* **2011**, *113*, 999–1016. [CrossRef] [PubMed]
30. Eather, N.; Bull, A.; Young, M.D.; Barnes, A.T.; Pollock, E.R.; Morgan, P.J. Fundamental movement skills: Where do girls fall short? A novel investigation of object-control skill execution in primary-school aged girls. *Prev. Med. Rep.* **2018**, *11*, 191–195. [CrossRef]
31. Navarro-Patón RLago-Ballesteros, J.; Arufe-Giráldez, V.; Sanmiguel-Rodríguez, A.; Lago-Fuentes, C.; Mecías-Calvo, M. Gender differences in motor competence in 5-year-old preschool children regarding relative age. *Int. J. Environ. Res. Public Health* **2021**, *18*, 3143. [CrossRef]
32. Morley, D.; Till, K.; Ogilvie, P.; Turner, G. Influences of gender and socioeconomic status on the motor proficiency of children in the UK. *Hum. Mov. Sci.* **2015**, *44*, 150–156. [CrossRef] [PubMed]
33. Cliff, D.P.; Okely, A.D.; Smith, L.M.; McKeen, K. Relationships between fundamental movement skills and objectively measured physical activity in preschool children. *Pediatric Exerc. Sci.* **2009**, *21*, 436–449. [CrossRef] [PubMed]
34. Hardy, L.L.; Reinten-Reynolds, T.; Espinel, P.; Zask, A.; Okely, A.D. Prevalence and correlates of low fundamental movement skill competency in children. *Pediatrics* **2012**, *130*, e390–e398. [CrossRef]
35. Latorre Román, P.Á.; Moreno del Castillo, R.; Lucena Zurita, M.; Salas Sánchez, J.; García-Pinillos, F.; Mora López, D. Physical fitness in preschool children: Association with sex, age and weight status. *Child Care Health Dev.* **2017**, *43*, 267–273. [CrossRef]
36. Dencker, M.; Thorsson, O.; Karlsson, M.K.; Lindén, C.; Eiberg, S.; Wollmer, P.; Andersen, L.B. Gender differences and determinants of aerobic fitness in children aged 8–11 years. *Eur. J. Appl. Physiol.* **2007**, *99*, 19–26. [CrossRef] [PubMed]
37. Amusa, L.O.; Goon, D.T.; Amey, A.K. Gender differences in neuromotor fitness of rural South African children. *Med. Sport* **2010**, *6*, 221–237.
38. Van Capelle, A.; Broderick, C.R.; van Doorn, N.; Ward, R.E.; Parmenter, B.J. Interventions to improve fundamental motor skills in pre-school aged children: A systematic review and meta-analysis. *J. Sci. Med. Sport* **2017**, *20*, 658–666. [CrossRef]
39. Peralta, L.R.; Mihrshahi, S.; Bellew, B.; Reece, L.J.; Hardy, L.L. Influence of School-Level Socioeconomic Status on Children's Physical Activity, Fitness, and Fundamental Movement Skill Levels. *J. Sch. Health* **2019**, *89*, 460–467. [CrossRef]
40. de Greeff, J.W.; Bosker, R.J.; Oosterlaan, J.; Visscher, C.; Hartman, E. Effects of physical activity on executive functions, attention and academic performance in preadolescent children: A meta-analysis. *J. Sci. Med. Sport* **2018**, *21*, 501–507. [CrossRef]
41. Prista, A.; Marques, A.; Maia, J. Relationship between physical activity, socioeconomic status, and physical fitness of 8–15-year-old youth from Mozambique. *Am. J. Hum. Biol.* **1997**, *9*, 449–457. [CrossRef]
42. Freitas, D.; Maia, J.M.; Beunen, G.; Claessens, A.; Thomis, M.; Marques, A.; Crespo, M.; Lefevre, J. Socio-economic status, growth, physical activity and fitness: The Madeira Growth Study. *Ann. Hum. Biol.* **2007**, *34*, 107–122. [CrossRef]
43. Hall, C.J.; Eyre, E.L.; Oxford, S.W.; Duncan, M.J. Relationships between motor competence, physical activity, and obesity in British preschool aged children. *J. Funct. Morphol. Kinesiol.* **2018**, *3*, 57. [CrossRef]
44. Donnelly, J.E.; Greene, J.L.; Gibson, C.A.; Smith, B.K.; Washburn, R.A.; Sullivan, D.K.; Williams, S.L. Physical Activity Across the Curriculum (PAAC): A randomized controlled trial to promote physical activity and diminish overweight and obesity in elementary school children. *Prev. Med.* **2009**, *49*, 336–341. [CrossRef]
45. Keller, B.A. State of the art reviews: Development of fitness in children: The influence of gender and physical activity. *Am. J. Lifestyle Med.* **2008**, *2*, 58–74. [CrossRef]
46. D'Haese, S.; Van Dyck, D.; De Bourdeaudhuij, I.; Deforche, B.; Cardon, G. The association between objective walkability, neighborhood socio-economic status, and physical activity in Belgian children. *Int. J. Behav. Nutr. Phys. Act.* **2014**, *11*, 1–8. [CrossRef]

47. National Norms And Standards For School Funding. Available online: https://www.education.gov.za/Portals/0/Documents/Legislation/Call%20for%20Comments/NATIONAL%20NORMS%20AND%20STANDARDS%20FOR%20SCHOOL%20FUNDING.pdf?ver=2008--03--05--104405--000 (accessed on 19 December 2021).
48. Eston, R.; Reilly, T. Kinanthropometry and Exercise Physiology Laboratory Manual: Tests, Procedures and Data. In *Physiology*; Routledge: Milton Park, UK, 2013; Volume 2.
49. Slaughter, M.H.; Lohman, T.G.; A Boileau, R.; A Horswill, C.; Stillman, R.J.; Van Loan, M.D.; A Bemben, D. Skinfold equations for estimation of body fatness in children and youth. *J. Hum. Biol.* **1988**, *60*, 709–723.
50. Reilly, J.J. Assessment of body fat percentage in infants and children. *Nutrition* **1988**, *14*, 821–825. [CrossRef]
51. Kriemler, S.; Puder, J.; Zahner, L.; Roth, R.; Meyer, U.; Bedogni, G. Estimation of percentage body fat in 6- to 13-year-old children by skinfold thickness, body mass index and waist circumference. *Br. J. Nutr.* **2010**, *104*, 1565–1572. [CrossRef]
52. Morrison, K.M.; Bugge, A.; El-Naaman, B.; Eisenmann, J.C.; Froberg, K.; Pfeiffer, K.A.; Andersen, L.B. Inter-Relationships Among Physical Activity, Body Fat, and Motor Performance in 6- to 8-Year-Old Danish Children. *Pediatr. Exerc. Sci.* **2012**, *24*, 199–209. [CrossRef] [PubMed]
53. Hassapidou, M.; Daskalou, E.; Tsofliou, F.; Tziomalos, K.; Paschaleri, A.; Pagkalos, I.; Tzotzas, T. Prevalence of overweight and obesity in preschool children in Thessaloniki, Greece. *Hormones* **2015**, *14*, 615–622. [CrossRef]
54. Teo, K.K.; Rafiq, T.; Anand, S.S.; Schulze, K.M.; Yusuf, S.; McDonald, S.D.; Wahi, G.; Abdalla, N.; Desai, D.; Atkinson, S.A.; et al. Associations of cardiometabolic outcomes with indices of obesity in children aged 5 years and younger. *PLoS ONE* **2019**, *14*, e0218816. [CrossRef]
55. Santos, S.; Severo, M.; Lopes, C.; Oliveira, A. Anthropometric Indices Based on Waist Circumference as Measures of Adiposity in Children. *Obesity* **2018**, *26*, 810–813. [CrossRef] [PubMed]
56. Nambiar, S.; Hughes, I.; Davies, P.S. Developing waist-to-height ratio cut-offs to define overweight and obesity in children and adolescents. *Public Health Nutr.* **2010**, *13*, 1566–1574. [CrossRef] [PubMed]
57. World Health Organization (WHO). The use and interpretation of anthropometry. *WHO Tech. Rep. Ser.* **1995**, *854*, 1–452.
58. Ulrich, D.A. *Test of Gross Motor Development*, 2nd ed.; Pro-Ed: Austin, TX, USA, 2000.
59. Foweather, L.; Knowles, Z.; Ridgers, N.; O'Dwyer, M.V.; Foulkes, J.D.; Stratton, G. Fundamental movement skills in relation to weekday and weekend physical activity in preschool children. *J. Sci. Med. Sport* **2015**, *18*, 691–696. [CrossRef]
60. Brien, W.O.; Belton, S.; Issartel, J. Fundamental movement skill proficiency amongst adolescent youth. *Phys. Educ. Sport Pedagog.* **2016**, *21*, 557–571. [CrossRef]
61. Bolger, L.E.; Bolger, L.A.; O'Neill, C.; Coughlan, E. Age and Sex Differences in Fundamental Movement Skills Among a Cohort of Irish School Children. *J. Mot. Learn. Dev.* **2018**, *6*, 81–100. [CrossRef]
62. Mukherjee, S.; Jamie, L.C.T.; Fong, L.H. Fundamental Motor Skill Proficiency of 6- to 9-Year-Old Singaporean Children. *Percept. Mot. Ski.* **2017**, *124*, 584–600. [CrossRef]
63. De Meester, A.; Stodden, D.; Goodway, J.; True, L.; Brian, A.; Ferkel, R.; Haerens, L. Identifying a motor proficiency barrier for meeting physical activity guidelines in children. *J. Sci. Med. Sport* **2018**, *21*, 58–62. [CrossRef]
64. Duncan, M.J.; Roscoe, C.M.; Noon, M.; Clark, C.; O'Brien, W.; Eyre, E. Run, jump, throw and catch: How proficient are children attending English schools at the fundamental motor skills identified as key within the school curriculum? *Eur. Phys. Educ. Rev.* **2020**, *26*, 814–826. [CrossRef]
65. Pienaar, A. Kinderkinetics: An investment in the total well-being of children. *S. Afr. J. Res. Sport Phys. Educ. Recreat.* **2009**, *31*, 49–67. [CrossRef]
66. Parızková, J.; Sedlak, P.; Dvorakova, H.; Lisá, L.; Bláha, P. Secular trends of adiposity and motor abilities in preschool children. *Obes. Weight. Loss Ther.* **2012**, *2*, 153. [CrossRef]
67. Ortega, F.B.; Cadenas-Sánchez, C.; Sanchez-Delgado, G.; Mora-Gonzalez, J.; Tellez, B.M.; Artero, E.G.; Castro-Piñero, J.; Labayen, I.; Chillón, P.; Löf, M.; et al. Systematic Review and Proposal of a Field-Based Physical Fitness-Test Battery in Preschool Children: The PREFIT Battery. *Sports Med.* **2015**, *45*, 533–555. [CrossRef]
68. Cadenas-Sanchez, C.; Martinez-Tellez, B.; Sanchez-Delgado, G.; Mora-Gonzalez, J.; Castro-Piñero, J.; Löf, M.; Ruiz, J.R.; Ortega, F.B. Assessing physical fitness in preschool children: Feasibility, reliability and practical recommendations for the PREFIT battery. *J. Sci. Med. Sport* **2016**, *19*, 910–915. [CrossRef]
69. Hair, J.F.; Black, W.C.; Babin, B.J.; Anderson, R.E. *Multivariate Data Analysis: Pearson New International Edition*; Pearson Education Limited: London, UK, 2014.
70. Cohen, J. *Statistical Power Analysis for the Behavioral Sciences*, 2nd ed.; Lawrence Erlbaum: Mahwah, NJ, USA, 1988.
71. Grissom, R.J.; Kim, J.J. *Effect Sizes for Research: Univariate and Multivariate Applications*; Routledge: Milton Park, UK, 2012.
72. Hintze, J. NCSS 2007; NCSS LLC: Kaysville, UT, USA, 2007; Available online: www.ncss.com (accessed on 16 September 2021).
73. Shen, A.; Bernabé, E.; Sabbah, W. Severe dental caries is associated with incidence of thinness and overweight among preschool Chinese children. *Acta Odontol. Scand.* **2019**, *78*, 203–209. [CrossRef] [PubMed]
74. Cecil, J.; Watt, P.; Murrie, I.S.L.; Wrieden, W.; Wallis, D.; Hetherington, M.; Bolton-Smith, C.; Palmer, C. Childhood obesity and socioeconomic status: A novel role for height growth limitation. *Int. J. Obes.* **2005**, *29*, 1199–1203. [CrossRef]
75. Bann, D.; Johnson, W.; Li, L.; Kuh, D.; Hardy, R. Socioeconomic inequalities in childhood and adolescent body-mass index, weight, and height from 1953 to 2015: An analysis of four longitudinal, observational, British birth cohort studies. *Lancet Public Health* **2018**, *3*, e194–e203. [CrossRef]

76. Badran, M.; Laher, I. Obesity in Arabic-Speaking Countries. *J. Obes.* **2011**, *2011*, 1–9. [CrossRef]
77. Addo, I.Y.; Brener, L.; Asante, A.D.; de Wit, J. Socio-cultural beliefs about an ideal body size and implications for risk of excess weight gain after immigration: A study of Australian residents of sub-Saharan African ancestry. *Ethn. Health* **2019**, *26*, 1209–1224. [CrossRef]
78. Choukem, S.-P.; Tochie, J.N.; Sibetcheu, A.T.; Nansseu, J.R.; Hamilton-Shield, J.P. Overweight/obesity and associated cardiovascular risk factors in sub-Saharan African children and adolescents: A scoping review. *Int. J. Pediatr. Endocrinol.* **2020**, *2020*, 6. [CrossRef]
79. Viner, R.M.; Haines, M.M.; Taylor, S.; Head, J.; Booy, R.; Stansfeld, S. Body mass, weight control behaviours, weight perception and emotional well being in a multiethnic sample of early adolescents. *Int. J. Obes.* **2006**, *30*, 1514–1521. [CrossRef] [PubMed]
80. Kruger, H.S.; Puoane, T.; Senekal, M.; Van Der Merwe, M.-T. Obesity in South Africa: Challenges for government and health professionals. *Public Health Nutr.* **2005**, *8*, 491–500. [CrossRef]
81. Puoane, T.; Fourie, J.M.; Shapiro, M.; Rosling, L.; Tshaka, N.C.; Oelefse, A. 'Big is beautiful'-an exploration with urban black community health workers in a South African township. *S. Afr. J. Clin. Nutr.* **2005**, *18*, 6–15. [CrossRef]
82. Bosire, E.N.; Cohen, E.; Erzse, A.; Goldstein, S.J.; Hofman, K.J.; Norris, S.A. 'I'd say I'm fat, I'm not obese': Obesity normalisation in urban-poor South Africa. *Public Health Nutr.* **2020**, *23*, 1515–1526. [CrossRef]
83. Marsh, H.W.; Hau, K.T.; Sung, R.Y.T.; Yu, C.W. Childhood obesity, gender, actual-ideal body image discrepancies, and physical self-concept in Hong Kong children: Cultural differences in the value of moderation. *Dev. Psychol.* **2007**, *43*, 647–662. [CrossRef] [PubMed]
84. Jones, A. Race, Socioeconomic Status, and Health during Childhood: A Longitudinal Examination of Racial/Ethnic Differences in Parental Socioeconomic Timing and Child Obesity Risk. *Int. J. Environ. Res. Public Health* **2018**, *15*, 728. [CrossRef]
85. Adkins, M.M.; Bice, M.R.; Dinkel, D.; Rech, J.P. Leveling the Playing Field: Assessment of Gross Motor Skills in Low Socioeconomic Children to their Higher Socioeconomic Counterparts. *Int. J. Kinesiol. Sports Sci.* **2017**, *5*, 28–34. [CrossRef]
86. Fu, Y.; Burns, R.D. Effect of an Active Video Gaming Classroom Curriculum on Helath-Related Fitness, School Day Step Counts, and Motivation in Sixth Graders. *J. Phys. Act. Health.* **2018**, *15*, 644–650. [CrossRef]
87. Tomaz, S.A.; Hinkley, T.; Jones, R.A.; Twine, R.; Kahn, K.; Norris, S.A.; Draper, C.E. Objectively Measured Physical Activity in South African Children Attending Preschool and Grade R: Volume, Patterns, and Meeting Guidelines. *Pediatr. Exerc. Sci.* **2020**, *32*, 150–156. [CrossRef] [PubMed]
88. Goodway, J.D.; Smith, D.W. Keeping all children healthy: Challenges to leading an active lifestyle for preschool children qualifying for at-risk programs. *Fam. Community Health* **2005**, *28*, 142–155. [CrossRef] [PubMed]
89. Gosselin, V.; Leone, M.; Laberge, S. Socioeconomic and gender-based disparities in the motor competence of school-age children. *J. Sports Sci.* **2021**, *39*, 341–350. [CrossRef]
90. Jones, R.A.; Riethmuller, A.; Hesketh, K.; Trezise, J.; Batterham, M.; Okely, A. Promoting Fundamental Movement Skill Development and Physical Activity in Early Childhood Settings: A Cluster Randomized Controlled Trial. *Pediatr. Exerc. Sci.* **2011**, *23*, 600–615. [CrossRef] [PubMed]
91. Dinkel, D.; Snyder, K.; Patterson, T.; Warehime, S.; Kuhn, M.; Wisneski, D. An exploration of infant and toddler unstructured outdoor play. *Eur. Early Child. Educ. Res. J.* **2019**, *27*, 257–271. [CrossRef]
92. Behrens, R.; Muchaka, P. Child Independent Mobility in South Africa: The Case of Cape Town and its Hinterland. *Glob. Stud. Child.* **2011**, *1*, 167–184. [CrossRef]
93. Larouche, R.; Oyeyemi, A.L.; Prista, A.; Onywera, V.; Akinroye, K.K.; Tremblay, M.S. A systematic review of active transportation research in Africa and the psychometric properties of measurement tools for children and youth. *Int. J. Behav. Nutr. Phys. Act.* **2014**, *11*, 129. [CrossRef]
94. Draper, C.E.; Tomaz, S.A.; Stone, M.; Hinkley, T.; Jones, R.A.; Louw, J.; Twine, R.; Kahn, K.; Norris, S. Developing Intervention Strategies to Optimise Body Composition in Early Childhood in South Africa. *BioMed Res. Int.* **2017**, *2017*, 1–13. [CrossRef]
95. Cook, C.J.; Howard, S.J.; Scerif, G.; Twine, R.; Kahn, K.; Norris, S.A.; Draper, C.E. Associations of physical activity and gross motor skills with executive function in preschool children from low-income South African settings. *Dev. Sci.* **2019**, *22*, e12820. [CrossRef] [PubMed]
96. VandenDriessche, J.B.; Vaeyens, R.; Vandorpe, B.; Lenoir, M.; Lefevre, J.; Philippaerts, R.M. Variation in sport participation, fitness and motor coordination with socioeconomic status among Flemish children. *Pediatric Exerc. Sci.* **2012**, *24*, 113–128. [CrossRef]
97. Sandercock, G.R.; Lobelo, F.; Correa-Bautista, J.E.; Tovar, G.; Cohen, D.D.; Knies, G.; Ramírez-Vélez, R. The Relationship between Socioeconomic Status, Family Income, and Measures of Muscular and Cardiorespiratory Fitness in Colombian Schoolchildren. *J. Pediatr.* **2017**, *185*, 81–87.e2. [CrossRef]
98. Haro, I.M.-D.; Mora-Gonzalez, J.; Cadenas-Sanchez, C.; Borras, P.A.; Benito, P.J.; Chiva-Bartoll, O.; Torrijos-Niño, C.; Samaniego-Sánchez, C.; Quesada-Granados, J.J.; Sánchez-Delgado, A.; et al. Higher socioeconomic status is related to healthier levels of fatness and fitness already at 3 to 5 years of age: The PREFIT project. *J. Sports Sci.* **2019**, *37*, 1327–1337. [CrossRef]
99. Wolfe, A.M.; Lee, J.A.; Laurson, K.R. Socioeconomic status and physical fitness in youth: Findings from the NHANES National Youth Fitness Survey. *J. Sports Sci.* **2020**, *38*, 534–541. [CrossRef]
100. Guedes, D.P.; Neto, J.M.; Lopes, V.P.; Silva, A. Health-Related Physical Fitness Is Associated with Selected Sociodemographic and Behavioral Factors in Brazilian School Children. *J. Phys. Act. Health* **2012**, *9*, 473–480. [CrossRef] [PubMed]

101. Macdonald, M.; McGuire, C.; Havighurst, R.J. Leisure Activities and the Socioeconomic Status of Children. *Am. J. Sociol.* **1949**, *54*, 505–519. [CrossRef]
102. Powell, L.M.; Slater, S.; Chaloupka, F.J.; Harper, D. Availability of Physical Activity-Related Facilities and Neighbourhood Demographic and Socioeconomic Charateristics: A National Study. *Am. J. Public Health* **2006**, *96*, 1676–1680. [CrossRef] [PubMed]
103. Micklesfield, L.; Pedro, T.; Twine, R.; Kinsman, J.; Pettifor, J.; Tollman, S.; Kahn, K.; Norris, S. Physical activity patterns and determinants in rural South African adolescents. *J. Sci. Med. Sport* **2012**, *15*, S251. [CrossRef]
104. Jayanthi, N.A.; Holt, J.D.B.; Labella, C.R.; Dugas, L.R. Socioeconomic Factors for Sports Specialization and Injury in Youth Athletes. *Sports Health* **2018**, *10*, 303–310. [CrossRef] [PubMed]
105. Lennox, A.; Pienaar, A.; Wilders, C. Physical fitness and the physical activity status of 15-year-old adolescents in a semi-urban community. *S. Afr. J. Res. Sport Phys. Educ. Recreat.* **2008**, *30*, 59–73. [CrossRef]
106. Bürgi, R.; Tomatis, L.; Murer, K.; de Bruin, E.D. Spatial physical activity patterns among primary school children living in neighbourhoods of varying socioeconomic status a cross-sectional study using accelerometry and Global Positioning System. *BMC Public Health* **2016**, *16*, 1–12. [CrossRef]
107. Ginsburg, K.R.; the Committee on Communications; the Committee on Psychosocial Aspects of Child and Family Health. The Importance of Play in Promoting Healthy Child Development and Maintaining Strong Parent-Child Bonds. *Pediatrics* **2007**, *119*, 182–191. [CrossRef]
108. Masters, R.S.; Maxwell, J.P. Implicit motor learning, reinvestment and movement disruption: What you don't know won't hurt you. In *Skill Acquisition in Sport*; Routledge: Milton Park, UK, 2004; pp. 231–252.
109. Kal, E.; Prosée, R.; Winters, M.; Van Der Kamp, J. Does implicit motor learning lead to greater automatization of motor skills compared to explicit motor learning? A systematic review. *PLoS ONE* **2018**, *13*, e0203591. [CrossRef]
110. Veraksa, A.; Aires, J.Q.; Leonov, S.; Musálek, M. The Vygotskian approach in physical education for early years. In *Vygotsky's Theory in Early Childhood Education and Research*; Routledge: Milton Park, UK, 2018; pp. 179–190.
111. Ponthieux, N.A.; Barker, D.G. Relationship between Socioeconomic Status and Physical Fitness Measures. *Res. Quarterly. Am. Assoc. Health Phys. Educ. Recreat.* **1965**, *36*, 464–472. [CrossRef]
112. Pavón, D.J. Socioeconomic status influences physical fitness in European adolescents independently of body fat and physical activity: The HELENA Study. *Nutr. Hosp.* **2010**, *25*, 311–316.
113. Coe, D.P.; Peterson, T.; Blair, C.; Schutten, M.C.; Peddie, H. Physical Fitness, Academic Achievement, and Socioeconomic Status in School-Aged Youth. *J. Sch. Health* **2013**, *83*, 500–507. [CrossRef]
114. Stastny, P.; Lehnert, M.; Croix, M.D.S.; Petr, M.; Svoboda, Z.; Maixnerova, E.; Varekova, R.; Botek, M.; Petrek, M.; Kocourkova, L.; et al. Effect of COL5A1, GDF5, and PPARA Genes on a Movement Screen and Neuromuscular Performance in Adolescent Team Sport Athletes. *J. Strength Cond. Res.* **2019**, *33*, 2057–2065. [CrossRef]
115. Chan, T.-F.; Poon, A.; Basu, A.; Addleman, N.R.; Chen, J.; Phong, A.; Byers, P.H.; Klein, T.E.; Kwok, P.-Y. Natural variation in four human collagen genes across an ethnically diverse population. *Genomics* **2008**, *91*, 307–314. [CrossRef] [PubMed]
116. Adamo, K.B.; Sheel, A.W.; Onywera, V.; Waudo, J.; Boit, M.; Tremblay, M.S. Child obesity and fitness levels among Kenyan and Canadian children from urban and rural environments: A KIDS-CAN Research Alliance Study. *Pediatr. Obes.* **2011**, *6*, e225–e232. [CrossRef] [PubMed]
117. Prista, A.; Maia, J.A.R.; Damasceno, A.; Beunen, G. Anthropometric indicators of nutritional status: Implications for fitness, activity, and health in school-age children and adolescents from Maputo, Mozambique. *Am. J. Clin. Nutr.* **2003**, *77*, 952–959. [CrossRef] [PubMed]
118. Tompsett, C.; Sanders, R.; Taylor, C.; Cobley, S. Pedagogical Approaches to and Effects of Fundamental Movement Skill Interventions on Health Outcomes: A Systematic Review. *Sports Med.* **2017**, *47*, 1795–1819. [CrossRef]
119. Katzmarzyk, P.; Malina, R.; Beunen, G. The contribution of biological maturation to the strength and motor fitness of children. *Ann. Hum. Biol.* **1997**, *24*, 493–505. [CrossRef] [PubMed]
120. Malina, R.M.; Bouchard, C.; Bar-Or, O. *Growth, Maturation, and Physical Activity*; Human Kinetics: Champaign, IL, USA, 2004.

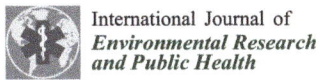

Article

Somatotype Profiles of Montenegrin Karatekas: An Observational Study

Jelena Slankamenac [1], Dusko Bjelica [2], Damjan Jaksic [1], Tatjana Trivic [1], Miodrag Drapsin [3], Sandra Vujkov [4], Toni Modric [5], Zoran Milosevic [1] and Patrik Drid [1,*]

[1] Faculty of Sport and Physical Education, University of Novi Sad, 21000 Novi Sad, Serbia; jelly.95@live.com (J.S.); jaksic_damjan@yahoo.com (D.J.); ttrivic@yahoo.com (T.T.); zoranaisns29@gmail.com (Z.M.)
[2] Faculty of Sports and Physical Education, University of Montenegro, 81400 Nikšić, Montenegro; montenegrosportmont@t-com.me
[3] Faculty of Medicine, University of Novi Sad, 21000 Novi Sad, Serbia; miodrag.drapsin@mf.uns.ac.rs
[4] College of Vocational Studies for the Education of Preschool Teachers and Sports Trainers, 24000 Subotica, Serbia; sandravujkov@vsovsu.rs
[5] Faculty of Kinesiology, University of Split, 21000 Split, Croatia; toni.modric@kifst.hr
* Correspondence: patrikdrid@gmail.com

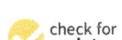

Citation: Slankamenac, J.; Bjelica, D.; Jaksic, D.; Trivic, T.; Drapsin, M.; Vujkov, S.; Modric, T.; Milosevic, Z.; Drid, P. Somatotype Profiles of Montenegrin Karatekas: An Observational Study. *Int. J. Environ. Res. Public Health* **2021**, *18*, 12914. https://doi.org/10.3390/ijerph182412914

Academic Editors: Francesco Campa and Gianpiero Greco

Received: 21 October 2021
Accepted: 30 November 2021
Published: 7 December 2021

Publisher's Note: MDPI stays neutral with regard to jurisdictional claims in published maps and institutional affiliations.

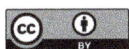

Copyright: © 2021 by the authors. Licensee MDPI, Basel, Switzerland. This article is an open access article distributed under the terms and conditions of the Creative Commons Attribution (CC BY) license (https://creativecommons.org/licenses/by/4.0/).

Abstract: Competitive karate activity involves numerous factors affecting performance in sport. Physical structure and somatotype is considered to be one of them. This study aimed to determine whether there are differences between karate athletes in five male and five female official weight categories in different anthropometric measurements and to determine the somatotype profiles of athletes divided by weight categories. This study consisted of a total of 27 male karate athletes (21.88 ± 4.66 years) and 24 female karate athletes (20.29 ± 3.14 years). Measurements were taken in April 2020. Athletes are classified into official weight categories according to World Karate Federation rules. Somatotypes were calculated using anthropometry. One-way analysis of variance and Tukey's post hoc tests were used for statistical analysis to compare group differences regarding weight categories. Anthropometric parameters were highest in the heaviest categories compared to lighter categories. All male subjects were endomorphic mesomorph, except for category <84 kg, which was endomorphic ectomorphs. Somatotype analysis of male categories found a difference between the <75 kg and <84 kg in endomorphy. In mesomorphy, there is no difference between categories. Perceiving ectomorphy, there is a significant difference between the first category and the >84 kg. Profiling female athletes, three different types of somatotypes were obtained concerning the weight category. The lightest weight category was predominantly endomorphic ectomorphs, and two weight categories were ectomorphic endomorphs (<61 kg and <68 kg), and the other two weight categories were endomorphic mesomorphs (<55 kg and >68 kg). Somatotype differences in the female karate athletes were observed only in the ectomorphy components, between <50 kg and <61 kg. The present study points to how the somatotypes profiles of karate athletes differ between weight categories.

Keywords: karate; kumite; weight categories; anthropometry; body composition; martial arts; combat sports

1. Introduction

The origin of karate remains hidden by opaque veil legends, but we still know that karate originates from the Far East, and it was widely practiced by the people who were followers of such different religions as Buddhism, Islam, Hinduism, and Taoism. It was first developed in Okinawa, Japan, in the 17th century when the Japanese took this island and prohibited the usage of all weapons [1]. It gained popularity after the Second World War. Karate is one of the most popular and widely practiced martial arts of today, and only in 2021 (Tokyo, Japan) had its appearance in the Olympic games. It is characterized by two distinguished competitive disciplines: *Kata* and *Kumite* (sports fight). *Kata* means form, and it is a predetermined series of offensive and defensive techniques and movements in standard order, versus one or more nonexistent opponents. Fundamental elements of the *Kata* technique involve rhythm, expressiveness, and *Kime* (a short isometric muscle contraction performed when a technique is finished) [2]. Karatekas that outreach the final are obligated to perform one *Tokui* (free-style *Kata*) and one *Shitei* (fixed *Kata* styles). Athletes have 60–80 s to complete the *Kata* [3]. *Kumite*, on the other hand, represents combat between two karate athletes under certain rules. Strikes are limited to determining areas: face, head, neck, chest, abdomen, side, and back. The duration of the *Kumite* match is 3 min for male and female senior athletes [3]. Judges score kicks and punches—*Ippon* (3 points), *Waza-ari* (2 points), and *Yuko* (1 point). Points are awarded when a technique is executed according to the following principle: good form, vigorous application, sporting attitude, awareness, correct distance, and good timing. *Kumite* competitors are divided into five weight categories for both males and females (<60 kg, <67 kg, <75 kg, <84 kg and >84 kg for males and <50 kg, <55 kg, <61 kg, <68 kg and >68 kg for females). Weight categories in karate and other combat sports can ensure fair competition by complementary opponents of similar body mass and stature [4].

One of the oldest questions in every sport is "what actually makes a successful athlete successful?" Morphological features play an important role in accomplishments in most sports. Body form provides a foundation for the improvement of movement technique and particular physical fitness. When selecting athletes in a particular sport, it is observed whether their physical characteristics fit with a "model" somatic pattern for that sport. That model is based on somatic patterns recorded in athletes who have systematically achieved the best results. Assessment of body composition consists of an assessment of the somatotype, which is based on the relationship between body fat and the lean body content, muscular development, skeleton robustness, and reciprocal ponderal index (height divided by the cube root of body weight) [5–8]. The most commonly used technique in somatotype assessment is the Heath and Carter method [9]. They emphasize that the somatotype is defined as representing the individual's present morphological conformation. Heath-Carter method is used primarily in its anthropometric form in practice, and it is best suited for sports science. Anthropometric measurements are objective and can show body shape, composition, and proportionality. The somatotype consists of three main components in relation to body height: endomorphy, mesomorphy, and ectomorphy [10]. Endomorphy is the first component, and it represents relative fatness or leanness. The second component is mesomorphy and this shows relative musculoskeletal development adjusted for height. Ectomorphy, the third component, is the relative linearity of the build [5]. The knowledge of these characteristics is most informative for coaches and athletes.

Very often, the physical structure is considered as one of the elements for high performance in many sports, as well as in competitive karate [11,12]. In karate, empirical experience states that the athlete's body height and longitudinal dimensions, such as arm and leg length, are some of the main advantages of karate athletes because these measures allow karatekas to raise their legs higher during the kick and they can fight from greater distances [13]. Comparing karate athletes with the general population, they are distinguished by muscular mass with enhanced transverse skeleton dimensionality and reduced adipose tissue. It is known that the body composition of athletes has a great impact on achieving top sports results. Up to date, several studies have dealt with somatotypes in male karate athletes [14–16]. However, there is a lack of evidence regarding female karate somatotype. With this in mind, anthropometric parameters were measured, and the somatotypes of both male and female Montenegrin karatekas were determined.

This study aimed to determine whether there are differences between karate athletes in five male and five female weight categories in different anthropometric measurements and to determine the somatotype profiles of athletes. The results of this study should provide a more specific outline of the morphological biotype best suited to the specific technical requirements for *Kumite* athletes of both genders.

2. Materials and Methods

2.1. Subjects

A total of 60 senior karate athletes from Montenegro participated in the National Championships in 2020. For the purpose of this study, we have chosen 51 karate athletes (black belt). According to the calculation, considering that the five weight categories are analyzed, the total sample size should be much larger. However, in this specific case, the total population is 60 competitors, so the classical formula cannot be applied. A cohort of 27 male (21.9 ± 4.7years) and 24 female karate athletes (20.3 ± 3.14 years) of a national level volunteered in this cross-sectional study. The subject sample included healthy, black belt karate senior athletes, with no prior injuries, minimum five year training experience and overall weekly training volume of over 20 h. Measurements were taken in April 2020. All testing procedures were conducted during the karate camp ahead of the National Championship held in Nikšić (Montenegro). Participants were divided into five official male categories <60 kg ($n = 5$), <67 kg ($n = 8$), <75 kg ($n = 6$), <84 kg ($n = 4$), and >84 kg ($n = 4$) and five female weight categories <50 kg ($n = 2$), <55 kg ($n = 7$), <61 kg ($n = 7$), <68 kg ($n = 6$), and >68 kg ($n = 2$) in accordance with their current body mass, age and gender [3]. All athletes were introduced to all of the testing procedures applied in the current research. All anthropometrical measurements were taken from the participants in the same position, in the morning hours (before breakfast), by the same two experienced graduated students of the Faculty for Sport and Physical Education, University of Montenegro. Informed written consent was acquired from each subject, and all procedures were executed and conducted according to the guidelines of the Declaration of Helsinki and approved by the Institutional Review Board of the Faculty of Sport and Physical Education University of Novi Sad, Serbia (Ref. No. 46-06-02/2020-1).

2.2. Anthropometrical Measurements

In order to determine somatotypes, ten required measurements were taken as follows: body height and body mass, bi-epicondylar breadths of humerus and femur, four skinfold measurements (triceps, supraspinal, subscapular, and medial calf), and two girths (arm and calf). Body height (cm) was determined using a Martin anthropometer (GPM, Bachenbülach, Switzerland); body mass (kg) was measured with an electronic scale (SECA, Hamburg, Germany) with a sensitivity level of 0.1 kg; skinfolds were taken on the right side of the body using a John Bull caliper (British Indicator Ltd., Weybridge, UK), accurate to 0.2 mm; circumference measurements (cm) were obtained with a steel measuring tape, and wrist girth and bi-epicondylar diameters of the femur and humerus (mm) were measured using a small spreading caliper (SiberHegner, Zurich, Switzerland). Somatotypes were determined using the Carter and Heath method [9].

2.3. Statistical Analysis

The data obtained are presented as standard deviation (±) and means. One-way analysis of variance (ANOVA) and Tukey's post hoc tests was used to compare group the differences by weight categories. Furthermore, the effect size (h2) was calculated. The level of significance was set at p-value < 0.05. SPSS statistics software was used to conduct analyses.

3. Results

The study involved 27 male and 24 female Montenegrin karate athletes. Anthropometric characteristics and somatotype parameters were measured and presented in tables and charts. Both males and females were divided into five weight categories (male: <60 kg, <67 kg, <75 kg, <84 kg and >84 kg; female: <50 kg, <55 kg, <61 kg, <68 kg and >68 kg). Anthropometric parameters increased within the weight category.

Statistically significant differences in male categories were found between the first category (<60 kg) in body height compared to the last three categories (<75 kg, <84 kg, and >84 kg). The highest athletes were in the <84 kg category. There was no significant difference found between groups in breadths of humerus and femur. In term of arm girths, there were differences between <60 kg, <67 kg and >84 kg. However, a difference between <60 kg and the last three categories (<75 kg, <84 kg, and >84 kg) in terms of calf circumference was found.

Measuring skinfolds, statistically significant differences were shown only between <84 kg and the first three groups (<60 kg, <67 kg, and <75 kg) in supraspinal skinfold. Other differences in skinfolds were not at a significant level (Table 1).

Table 1. Differences between weight categories of male karatekas.

Male Variable	−60 [a] (n = 5) M ± SD	−67 [b] (n = 8) M ± SD	−75 [c] (n = 6) M ± SD	−84 [d] (n = 4) M ± SD	+84 [e] (n = 4) M ± SD	Statistics
Body height (cm)	168 ± 8.2	176.6 ± 7.2	183.9 ± 2.7 [a]	185.1 ± 3.5 [a]	184.8 ± 6.4 [a]	$F = 7.16, p = 0.001, \eta^2 = 0.57$
Breadths						
Humerus (cm)	7.3 ± 1	7.1 ± 0.6	7.6 ± 0.9	7.3 ± 0.2	7.4 ± 0.5	$F = 0.31, p = 0.869, \eta^2 = 0.05$
Femur (cm)	9.2 ± 1	9.6 ± 0.4	10.2 ± 1	10.3 ± 0.5	10.1 ± 0.3	$F = 1.98, p = 0.133, \eta^2 = 0.26$
Girths						
Arm (cm)	23.5 ± 2.8	25.9 ± 1.1	27.4 ± 1.2	26.4 ± 1.5	29.2 ± 1.8 [a,b]	$F = 7.32, p = 0.001, \eta^2 = 0.57$
Calf (cm)	34.2 ± 3	36.6 ± 1.4	38.1 ± 2 [a]	39.1 ± 1.7 [a]	40.5 ± 2 [a,b]	$F = 6.59, p = 0.001, \eta^2 = 0.55$
Skinfolds						
Triceps (mm)	9.4 ± 3.9	8.2 ± 2.4	6.3 ± 1.3	9.2 ± 1.2	8.4 ± 5.3	$F = 0.90, p = 0.479, \eta^2 = 0.14$
Supraspinale (mm)	6.4 ± 1.8	7.5 ± 2.2	6.6 ± 2.2	14.9 ± 3.6 [a,b,c]	11.1 ± 4.8	$F = 7.33, p = 0.001, \eta^2 = 0.57$
Subscapular (mm)	7.4 ± 1.1	8.8 ± 1.3	8.3 ± 1	8.6 ± 1.1	10.8 ± 2.4	$F = 3.53, p = 0.230, \eta^2 = 0.39$
Calf (mm)	9.5 ± 4.5	8.5 ± 2.6	6.7 ± 1.8	11 ± 2.6	9.5 ± 3.9	$F = 1.32, p = 0.293, \eta^2 = 0.19$
Somatotypes						
Endomorphy	2.3 ± 0.6	2.3 ± 0.6	1.9 ± 0.4	3.4 ± 1 [c]	2.8 ± 1.2	$F = 2.21, p = 0.100, \eta^2 = 0.29$
Mesomorphy	3.8 ± 1.5	3.7 ± 1.1	4 ± 1.2	2.5 ± 1.6	4.4 ± 1	$F = 0.32, p = 0.857, \eta^2 = 0.06$
Ectomorphy	3.9 ± 1.3	3.1 ± 1.1	3.2 ± 0.3	2.6 ± 0.7	1.8 ± 1.2 [a]	$F = 2.81, p = 0.051, \eta^2 = 0.34$

Legend: M—Mean; SD—standard deviation; different from: [a]—<60; [b]—<67; [c]—<75; [d]—<84; [e]—>85; significant differences in bold.

Somatotype analysis of male categories found a difference between the <75 kg and <84 kg in endomorphy. In mesomorphy, there is no difference between the categories. Perceiving ectomorphy, there is a significant difference between the first category and the >84 kg. All male subjects were endomorphic mesomorph, except for category <84 kg, which was endomorphic ectomorphs (Figure 1).

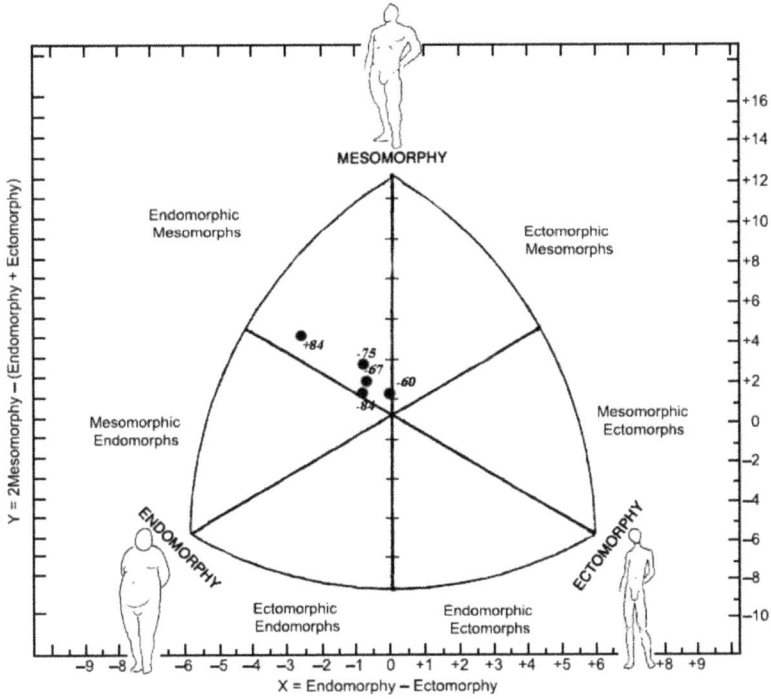

Figure 1. Somatochart of male karate athletes by weight categories.

In the female groups, body height increased in relation to the weight category and differed significantly between <50 kg, <55 kg, <61 kg, and the heaviest group (>68 kg), and between the first two (<50 kg, and <55 kg) and <68 kg. The breadth of the humerus shows a difference between >68 kg and all of the other groups (<50 kg, <55 kg, <61 kg, <68 kg). The only difference in the breadth of the femur is between the lightest (<50 kg) and the heaviest (>68 kg) category. Measuring arm circumference, there is one difference, between the <50 kg and >68 kg categories. Additionally, there is one difference between the groups in the circumference of the calf, between <50 kg and >68 kg. The categories did not differ significantly in terms of the thickness of the skin folds (Table 3).

Table 2. Differences between weight categories of female karatekas.

Female Variable	−50 [a] (n = 2) M ± SD	−55 [b] (n = 7) M ± SD	−61 [c] (n = 7) M ± SD	−68 [d] (n = 6) M ± SD	+68 [e] (n = 2) M ± SD	Statistics
Body height (cm)	161.5 ± 6.4	162.8 ± 4.7	163.8 ± 2.9	171.5 ± 5.5 [b,c]	181.0 ± 0 [a,b,c]	$F = 9.66, p = 0.000,$ $\eta^2 = 0.67$
Breadths						
Humerus (cm)	5.6 ± 0.6	6.1 ± 0.2	6 ± 0.2	6.3 ± 0.9	7.8 ± 0.4 [a,b,c,d]	$F = 6.23, p = 0.002,$ $\eta^2 = 0.57$
Femur (cm)	7 ± 2.8	8.9 ± 0.2	8.3 ± 0.9	9.2 ± 0.9	10.5 ± 0.7 [a]	$F = 3.99, p = 0.016,$ $\eta^2 = 0.46$
Girths						
Arm (cm)	21.6 ± 2.8	23.5 ± 1.1	23.5 ± 0.9	23.8 ± 0.6	26.7 ± 3.7 [a]	$F = 3.86, p = 0.018,$ $\eta^2 = 0.45$
Calf (cm)	32.4 ± 0.1	35.1 ± 1.6	35.9 ± 1.4	36.8 ± 1.4	37.9 ± 3 [a]	$F = 4.49, p = 0.010,$ $\eta^2 = 0.49$

Table 3. Differences between weight categories of female karatekas.

Female	−50 [a] (n = 2)	−55 [b] (n = 7)	−61 [c] (n = 7)	−68 [d] (n = 6)	+68 [e] (n = 2)	Statistics
			Skinfolds			
Triceps (mm)	10.4 ± 2.5	11.9 ± 2.2	14.1 ± 3.9	11.7 ± 1.1	10 ± 2.6	$F = 1.53, p = 0.234, \eta^2 = 0.24$
Supraspinale (mm)	13 ± 5.6	7.1 ± 2.1	12.8 ± 6.4	13.7 ± 5.2	9.6 ± 6.2	$F = 1.82, p = 0.167, \eta^2 = 0.28$
Subscapular (mm)	8.3 ± 2	9 ± 1.6	11.2 ± 3.8	11.5 ± 5.3	10.2 ± 1.6	$F = 0.67, p = 0.622, \eta^2 = 0.12$
Calf (mm)	10.8 ± 1.5	12.7 ± 3.4	13 ± 2.5	14.1 ± 3.7	11.3 ± 1.3	$F = 0.66, p = 0.628, \eta^2 = 0.12$
			Somatotypes			
Endomorphy	3.4 ± 0.3	2.9 ± 0.6	3.9 ± 1	3.6 ± 1.1	2.8 ± 1.1	$F = 1.43, p = 0.264, \eta^2 = 0.23$
Mesomorphy	1.2 ± 1.9	3.4 ± 0.9	2.8 ± 0.8	2.9 ± 0.8	4.6 ± 0.5 [a]	$F = 3.78, p = 0.020, \eta^2 = 0.44$
Ectomorphy	4.1 ± 0 [c]	2.7 ± 1	2 ± 0.7	2.5 ± 0.9	2.6 ± 1	$F = 2.39, p = 0.087, \eta^2 = 0.34$

Legend: M—Mean; SD—standard deviation; different from: [a]—<50; [b]—<55; [c]—<61; [d]—<68; [e]—>68; significant differences in bold.

The somatochart showed that the lightest weight category was predominantly endomorphic ectomorphs. Two weight categories were ectomorphic endomorphs (<61 kg and <68 kg), and the other two weight categories were endomorphic mesomorphs (<55 kg and >68 kg). Somatotype differences in the female karate athletes were observed in the ectomorphy components, between <50 kg and <61 kg, and in mesomorphy between <50 kg and >68 kg. (Figure 2).

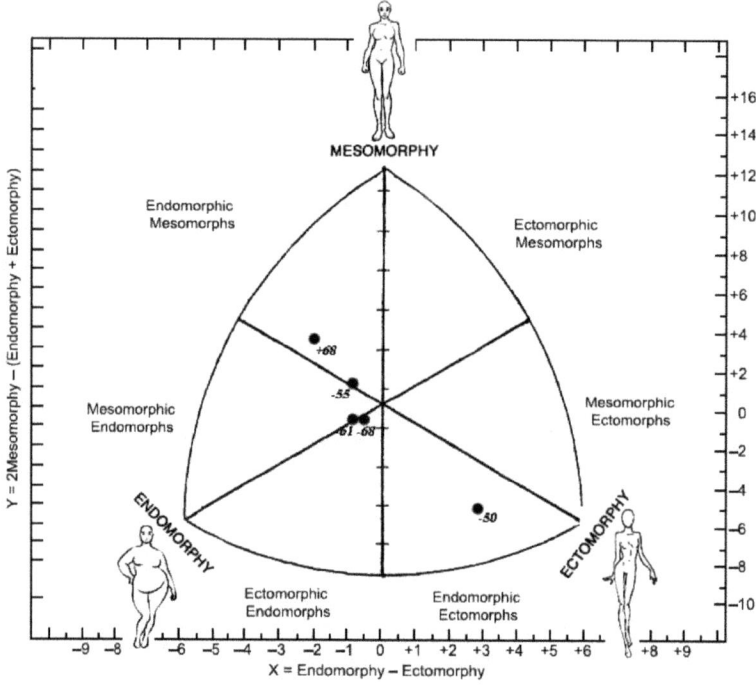

Figure 2. Somatochart of female karate athletes by weight categories.

4. Discussion

Accomplishment in most sports depends on the physical, physiological, psychological, and social characteristics of the athlete [17]. This study is focused on physical characteristics of karatekas, and determining whether there is a difference in these characteristics between Montenegrin karatekas in different weight categories.

The somatotype profiles of male and female Montenegrin karate athletes were evaluated in relation to different weight categories. Study results have indicated several differences in somatotype for the female group and some anthropometric characteristics throughout weight categories for both female and male groups of observed karate athletes. Somatotypes of male karatekas were mostly homogeneous. The obtained results showed the predominance of endomorphic mesomorphs, except for athletes in the <84 kg category, who were endomorphic ectomorphs. In contrast to our finding, some other recent studies found dominantly mesomorphic somatotypes in male karate athletes [18,19]. A higher mesomorphy component is significant in that increased muscle mass can be considered as an important benefit for athletes facing severe physical confrontation during training and competition, while increased fat mass reflected in endomorphism may prove useful in affecting absorption and dispersing such forces [20,21].

On the other hand, female karate athletes' results showed different types of somatotypes. Profiling female athletes, three different types of somatotypes in relation to weight category were obtained. Female categories show that the lightest weight category was predominantly endomorphic ectomorphs. Two weight categories were ectomorphic endomorphs (<61 kg and <68 kg), and the other two weight categories were endomorphic mesomorphs (<55 kg and >68 kg). This finding is in accordance with other studies that also examined anthropometric characteristics. Fritzsche and Raschka [14] state that the karatekas who practice *Kata* are exhibit more endomorphs characteristics and *Kumite* athletes take more ectomorph positions in somatocharts.

Karate athletes are characterized by a low percentage of fat tissue and a harmonic body constitution. However, different nationalities have different percentages of fat tissue [22]. A review of data from the literature discovered that elite karatekas are ectomorphic mesomorphs with a small amount of adipose tissue [23–25]. Prominent vertical skeletal development among top-level karatekas is the most influential anthropometric feature [23]. Controlling body composition is obligatory to clarify an athlete's best weight category [26].

In the present study, statistically significant differences in male categories were found between the first two categories in body height compared to the last three categories. In the female groups, body height increased concerning the weight category and differed significantly between <50 kg, <55 kg, <61 kg, and the heaviest group, and in between the first two and <68 kg. Gloc et al. [26] obtained the results which proposed that taller karate athletes with a higher percentage of muscular mass had a better outcome. Morphological characteristics also influence specific motor skills in junior karate athletes [27]. Analysis of bone diameters showed no significant differences in male categories, and in female categories, there are differences in the humerus breadth between the heaviest and all of the other groups; femur breadth was different between the lightest and the heaviest weight category. Azary and Izadi [28] stated that elite karatekas have longer lower limbs compared to non-elite athletes, despite their similarity in body height. They imply that Iranian karatekas have a higher skelic index than Italian athletes. Throughout karate sparring, various techniques are executed, and all of them require explosiveness and high speed to perform. The athletes with longer longitudinal dimensions seem to possess a particular superiority for acquiring points before the opponent, and they are able to use longer limb length to get the upper hand facing the opponent in combat [29]. Skinfolds differed significantly between groups, neither in the male nor the female categories, except between <84 kg and the first three groups in the supraspinal skinfold in male categories.

According to Przybylski et al. [30], the most significant qualificator factor for success in performing karate for each gender appears to be well-built strength based on the morphology of the limbs. In the current study, both male and female karatekas in the heaviest weight category differed significantly from the lighter categories in terms of anthropometric values.

One of the study limitations is presented by the relatively small number of athletes per each weight category. More athletes per each weight group could provide more detailed information regarding somatotypes in karate. Further investigation should be aimed on the dominant techniques typically used within categories and acquiring better insight into whether there is difference in the specific techniques that are used in relation to specific physical characteristics. Furthermore, it could be observed, additionally, whether specific techniques applied occur throughout various weight categories.

National level *Kumite* athletes of both genders in all weight categories were categorized by their physical characteristics in somatotypes in this study. Practicing karate seems to produce general morphological adaptation to the training process. Further studies are needed in order to investigate potential long-term adaptation in terms of the experience of athletes (i.e., national vs. international karatekas), as well as differences in somatotypes between *Kata* and *Kumite* athletes for both genders.

5. Conclusions

The findings of the study regarding somatotypes and anthropometric characteristics throughout various weight categories in karate should provide important information regarding future training processes, testing, as well as for the identification and selection of karate athletes. There are very few differences between karatekas in different weight categories. Differences were found between the heaviest and lighter categories in terms of body height, breadths, and girths in both male and female categories. There were no differences in the thickness of skin folds. Female categories show heterogeneous somatotypes, but the only significant difference was in ectomorphy between <50 kg and <61 kg. Male groups have similar somatotypes. Most of them were endomorphic mesomorphs. Significant differences between males were found in endomorphy (<67 kg and <84 kg) and in ectomorphy (<60 kg and >85 kg). By studying these characteristics, scientists can give specific details on the functional and morphological somatotype best suited for any sport. The present study could be significant for profiling and selecting karate athletes based on gender, age, and weight categories.

Author Contributions: Conceptualization, D.B., Z.M. and P.D.; Data curation, J.S., D.J., T.T., M.D. and S.V.; Formal analysis, D.J. and P.D.; Funding acquisition, D.B., and Z.M.; Investigation, J.S., D.J., T.T. and S.V.; Methodology, D.J. and P.D.; Project administration, T.M. and J.S.; Resources, P.D.; Software, D.J.; Supervision, D.B., Z.M. and P.D.; Validation, T.T. and T.M.; Visualization, D.J.; Writing—original draft, J.S., S.V. and P.D.; Writing—review & editing, J.S., D.B., D.J., T.T., M.D., S.V., T.M., Z.M. and P.D. All authors have read and agreed to the published version of the manuscript.

Funding: This work has been supported by the Serbian Ministry of Education, Science, and Technological Development (179011) and Provincial Secretariat for Higher Education and Scientific Research (142-451-2094).

Institutional Review Board Statement: The study was conducted according to the guidelines of the Declaration of Helsinki, and approved by the Institutional Review Board (or Ethics Committee) of University of Novi Sad, Serbia (Ref. No. 46-06-02/2020-1).

Informed Consent Statement: Informed consent was obtained from all subjects involved in the study.

Data Availability Statement: The data presented in this study are available on request from the corresponding author.

Conflicts of Interest: The authors declare that the research was conducted in the absence of any commercial or financial relationships that could be construed as a potential conflict of interest.

References

1. Chaabene, H.; Hachana, Y.; Franchini, E.; Mkaouer, B.; Chamari, K. Physical and Physiological Profile of Elite Karate Athletes. *Sports Med.* **2012**, *42*, 829–843. [CrossRef]
2. Doria, C.; Veicsteinas, A.; Limonta, E.; Maggioni, M.A.; Aschieri, P.; Eusebi, F.; Fanò, G.; Pietrangelo, T. Energetics of karate (kata and kumite techniques) in top-level athletes. *Eur. J. Appl. Physiol.* **2009**, *107*, 603–610. [CrossRef]
3. World Karate Federation (WKF): Kata and Kumite Competition Rules [Version Effective from 1.1.2020; Online]. Available online: https://www.wkf.net/pdf/WKF_Competition%20Rules_2020_EN.pdf (accessed on 1 October 2021).
4. Langan-Evans, C.; Close, G.L.; Morton, J.P. Making weight in combat sports. *Strength Cond. J.* **2011**, *33*, 25–39. [CrossRef]
5. Malina, R.; Bouchard, C.; Bar-Or, O. *Growth, Maturation, and Physical Activity*, 2nd ed.; Human Kinetics: Champaign, IL, USA, 2004.
6. Charzewski, J.; Glaz, A.; Kuzmicki, S. Somatotype characteristics of elite European wrestlers. *Biol. Sport* **1991**, *8*, 213–221.
7. Farmosi, I. Body-composition, somatotype and some motor performance of judoists. *J. Sports Med.* **1980**, *20*, 431–434.
8. Sklad, M.; Krawezyk, B.; Majle, B. Body build factors and body components in Greco-Roman and free-style wrestlers. *Biol. Sport* **1995**, *12*, 101–105.
9. Heath, B.H.; Carter, J.E. A modified somatotype method. *Am. J. Phys. Antropol.* **1967**, *27*, 54–74. [CrossRef]
10. Carter, J.E.; Heath, B.H. *Somatotyping. Development and Applications*; Cambridge University Press: New York, NY, USA, 1990.
11. Koropanovski, N.; Vujkov, S.; Jovanovic, S. Success factors for competitive karate. In *Science and Medicine in Combat Sports*; Drid, P., Ed.; Nova Publishers: New York, NY, USA, 2017; pp. 213–248.
12. Cinarli, F.S.; Kafkas, M.E. The effect of somatotype characters on selected physical performance parameters. *Phys. Educ. Stud.* **2019**, *23*, 279–287. [CrossRef]
13. Katić, R.; Blažević, S.; Krstulović, S.; Mulić, R. Morphological Structures of Elite Karatekas and Their Impact on Technical and Fighting Efficiency. *Coll. Antropol.* **2005**, *29*, 79–84.
14. Fritzsche, J.; Raschka, C. Sports anthropological investigations on somatotypology of elite karateka. *Anthropol. Anz.* **2007**, *65*, 317–329. [CrossRef]
15. Sterkowicz-Przybycien, K.L. Body Composition and Somatotype of the Top Polish Male Karate Contestants. *Biol. Sports* **2010**, *27*, 195–201. [CrossRef]
16. Pieter, W. Body Build of Elite Junior Taekwondo Athletes. *Acta Kinesiol. Univ. Tartu.* **2008**, *13*, 99–106. [CrossRef]
17. Catikkas, F.; Kurt, C.; Atalag, O. Kinanthropometric Attributes of Young Male Combat Sports Athletes. *Coll. Antropol.* **2013**, *37*, 1365–1368.
18. Shariat, A.; Shaw, B.S.; Kargarfard, M.; Shaw, I.; Lam, E.T.C. Kinanthropometric attributes of elite male judo, karate and taekwondo athletes. *Rev. Bras. Med. Esporte* **2017**, *23*, 260–263. [CrossRef]
19. Blerim, S.; Zarko, K.; Visar, G.; Agron, A.; Egzon, S. Differences in Anthropometrics Characteristics, Somatotype and Motor Skill in Karate and Non-Athletes. *Sport Sci. Health* **2017**, *7*, 108–111. [CrossRef]
20. Zbigniew, B.; Dariusz, G.; Elzbieta, H.W.; Sergejs, S. Anthropometric profile and anaerobic capacity of martial arts and combat sports athletes. *Ido Mov. Cult. J. Martial Arts Anthrop.* **2016**, *16*, 55–59.
21. Faraji, H.; Nikookheslat, S.D.; Fatollahi, S.; Alizadeh, M. Physical and Physiological Profile of Elite Iranian Karate Athletes. *Int. J. Appl. Exer. Physiol.* **2017**, *5*, 35–44.
22. Zombra, Ž. Differences in body composition between karate athletes and non-athletes. *Sport Sci. Pract. Asp.* **2018**, *15*, 31–36.
23. Giampietro, M.; Pujia, A.; Bertini, I. Anthropometric features and body composition of young athletes practicing karate at a high and medium competitive level. *Acta Diabetol.* **2003**, *40*, 145–148. [CrossRef] [PubMed]
24. Pieter, W.; Bercades, T.L. Somatotype of national elite combative sport athletes. *Braz. J. Biomot.* **2009**, *3*, 99–103.
25. Mendes, S.H.; Tritto, A.C.; Guilherme, J.P.L.; Solis, M.Y.; Vieira, D.E.; Franchini, E.; Lancha, A.H., Jr.; Artioli, G.G. Effect of rapid weight loss on performance in combat sport male athletes: Does adaptation to chronic weight cycling play a role? *Br. J. Sports Med.* **2013**, *47*, 1155–1160. [CrossRef]
26. Gloc, D.; Plewa, M.; Nowak, Z. The effects of kyokushin karate training on the anthropometry and body composition of advanced female and male practitioners. *J. Combat. Sports Martial Arts* **2012**, *3*, 36–71. [CrossRef]
27. Rakita, D.; Rakonjac, D.; Vukadinović-Jurišić, M.; Obradović, J. The influence of morphological characteristics on the specific motor skills of junior-age karate athletes. *Exerc. Qual. Life* **2018**, *10*, 43–49. [CrossRef]
28. Azari, H.; Izadi, M. Physical and physiological profile of Iranian world-class karate athlete. *Biomed. Hum. Kinet.* **2017**, *9*, 115–123.
29. Noorul, H.R.; Pieter, W.; Erie, Z.Z. Physical fitness of recreational adolescent taekwondo athletes. *Braz. J. Biomot.* **2008**, *2*, 230–240.
30. Przybylski, P.; Janiak, A.; Szewczyk, P.; Wielinski, D.; Domaszewska, K. Morphological and Motor Fitness Determinants of Shotokan Karate Performance. *Int. J. Environ. Res. Public Health* **2021**, *18*, 4423. [CrossRef] [PubMed]

Article

Body Size Measurements and Physical Performance of Youth Female Judo Athletes with Differing Menarcheal Status

Marina Saldanha da Silva Athayde [1,*], Rafael Lima Kons [1], David Hideyoshi Fukuda [2] and Daniele Detanico [1]

1. Laboratory, Center of Sports, Federal University of Santa Catarina, Florianópolis 88040, SC, Brazil; rafakons0310@gmail.com (R.L.K.); danieledetanico@gmail.com (D.D.)
2. Institute of Exercise Physiology and Rehabilitation Science, University of Central Florida, Orlando, FL 32816, USA; David.Fukuda@ucf.edu
* Correspondence: marinasaldanha.dsa@gmail.com; Tel.: +55-48-3721-8530

Abstract: *Purpose:* To compare body size measurements and physical performance among female youth judo athletes with differing menarcheal status and to identify indicators of physical performance in post-menarcheal girls. *Methods:* Nineteen young female judo athletes (age 13.9 ± 2.3 years) were divided into a pre-menarche ($n = 7$) and a post-menarche ($n = 12$) group. The athletes were evaluated through neuromuscular tests, including standing long jump (SLJ), medicine ball throw (MBT), and handgrip strength (HGS), and judo-specific assessments, including the Special Judo Fitness Test (SJFT) and the Judogi Grip Strength Test ($JGST_{ISO}$). Furthermore, years of experience in judo and the age at menarche were determined. *Results:* The main results showed higher performance for the post-menarche group for most variables ($p < 0.05$) compared to the pre-menarche group. A multiple linear regression analysis demonstrated that age at menarche, chronological age, and body mass explained close to 70% of $JGST_{ISO}$, while training experience, chronological age, and age at menarche explained close to 59% of SLJ. Additionally, chronological age and age at menarche explained 40% of MBT, and chronological age and height explained 52% of HGS. *Conclusions:* Age at menarche and somatic growth variables explained moderate proportions of the variance of physical performance, thereby providing evidence that these parameters are the primary indicators of physical performance in young female judo athletes.

Keywords: somatic maturity; puberty; combat sports; physical performance; young athletes

1. Introduction

Adolescence corresponds to the transition period between childhood and adulthood, during which several important biological manifestations occur, such as peak height velocity (PHV), peak weight velocity, sexual maturation, and, specifically for girls, menarche [1]. The range of variability in somatic and biological maturation among individuals of the same chronological age is large and is especially pronounced in adolescents [2]. When considering girls during this period, there is increased production of the estrogen hormone, responsible for stimulating growth and breast development [1], which is usually related to the first menstrual period (menarche) following PHV and considered an indication of biological maturation [3].

The current literature contains several studies on the effects of somatic maturity and growth on physical performance in young male athletes from team sports [4–7]. Most recently, studies have investigated the role of growth and maturity status on physical performance in young male judo athletes [8–12]. Years of formal judo training, growth, and somatic maturity can predict physical performance, when generalized upper and lower limb strength assessments (e.g., medicine ball throw test, handgrip strength, and jump tests) [8,10] and judo-specific tests (e.g., Special Judo Fitness Test and Judogi Grip Strength Test) [8] are considered. Moreover, Giudicelli et al. [11] found a positive relationship between maturity status and handgrip strength test as well as aerobic performance in young male judo athletes, even when chronological age and body mass were controlled. Thus, bearing in mind that judo athletes demand high levels of strength-related performance in the upper and lower limbs and both the aerobic and the anaerobic energy pathways [13], it is essential for coaches to understand the role of maturation during adolescence.

Many young female athletes are now involved in high-level judo competitions. For example, 223 female judo athletes from all continents participated in the 2019 World Cadet Judo Championship (under 18, U18), and 223 in the 2019 World Junior Judo Championship (U21) [14]. However, no studies investigating the effects of maturation on physical performance specifically in young female judo athletes have been conducted. It is known that girls present different somatic and physiological characteristics than boys due to variations in the timing and tempo of the maturation process [3,15] and, consequently, performance-related characteristics. A recent study with basketball players verified that girls with late maturity status (measured by the onset of menarche) tended to have less experience in the sport [16]. This study also found that body mass and adiposity were the highest predictors for all basketball performance indicators.

In individual sports, such as rhythmic gymnastics, Camargo et al. [17] found that there was an increase in the body fat percentage, fat mass, and fat-free mass 2 years after PHV and the occurrence of menarche. Furthermore, Pinto et al. [18] verified that girls in more advanced maturation stages presented higher values of growth indicators (weight and height) and power output of the upper limbs (through the medicine ball test). However, in individual sports of an intermittent nature requiring high-intensity actions, such as judo, these aspects are not yet fully known, in particular in relation to the physical demands of judo athletes, such as generic and judo-specific assessments.

Understanding the role of biological maturity (e.g., menarche), somatic growth measures (e.g., body size), and training experience in physical performance and their contribution in young female judo athletes can help coaches to design appropriate and individual training programs with consideration of biological development during adolescence. Thus, the purpose of this study was to compare body size measurements and physical performance among youth female judo athletes at different menarcheal statuses (pre- and post-menarche) in addition to identifying indicators of physical performance in post-menarche girls. We hypothesized that post-menarcheal girls are advanced in the growth process and consequently present higher physical performance.

2. Methods
2.1. Participants

Nineteen young female judo athletes (age 13.9 ± 2.3 years, range 10.9–17.0 years), purple ($n = 10$) and brown belts ($n = 9$), were divided into two groups: pre-menarche ($n = 7$) and post-menarche ($n = 12$). The athletes who participated in the study were from southern Brazil (Santa Catarina) and primarily of Portuguese ethnicity. The sample size was determined a priori using the GPower 3.1 software, taking as references a probability of 0.05 (minimum error type I), statistical power of 0.8 (minimum error type II), and effect size of 0.5 (mean effect). Thus, the minimum sample size was 21 participants. However, we were able to evaluate 19 athletes representing 48.7% of female athletes who participated in the competition in 2021, considering the age range of this study in the local federation ($n = 39$ athletes).

All athletes trained regularly with technical–tactical training occurring 2–3 times per week during the evaluation period, competed at the state and/or national levels, and had been engaged in formal training for at least 2 years. The girls reported no musculoskeletal disorders or injuries that would influence their maximal physical performance during the assessments. They were in the preparatory phase and therefore not in a period of rapid weight loss. All participants and responsible parties (parents and coaches/trainers) received a detailed verbal explanation of the purpose, methods, and potential risks/benefits of the study, followed by the completion of a written informed consent form. This study was approved by the Research Ethics Committee of the local university, in accordance with the Declaration of Helsinki.

2.2. Design

The athletes' assessments were performed during two afternoon testing visits separated by 48 h. During the first testing visit, an interview to determine the years of judo experience and age at menarche, anthropometric measurements (body mass and height), and neuromuscular tests (standing long jump test, medicine ball throw test, and handgrip strength test) were conducted. The physical tests were separated by 20 min intervals. At the second testing visit, the young judo athletes were submitted to sport-specific tests, including the Special Judo Fitness Test (SJFT) and the Judogi Grip Isometric Strength Test ($JGST_{ISO}$), separated by a 30 min recovery interval.

2.3. Determination of Menarcheal Status, Chronological Age, and Training Experience

Chronological age was calculated to the nearest 0.1 year by subtracting the date of birth from the date of testing. The number of years of formal training in judo was self-reported by the girls and/or their parents. Age at menarche was obtained through an individual interview with the girls by a female researcher; 12 athletes were determined to be post-menarche and 7 athletes pre-menarche. The body mass was measured using a digital scale Toledo® (0.1 kg accuracy), and height was assessed using a stadiometer scale of 0.1 cm accuracy.

3. Generic Tests

3.1. Standing Long Jump Test

For the standing long jump test, we followed the protocol used by Detanico et al. [8]. The girls performed the standing long jump test starting from a standing position by swinging their arms and flexing their knees to provide maximal forward drive. Before the assessment, the participants performed a familiarization/warm-up of 5 min of jogging, followed by 30 s of hopping, and 5 submaximal standing long jumps. A take-off line was drawn on the ground, and the measurement of the jump length was determined using a metric tape measure (Lufkin, L716MAGCME; Apex Group, Sparks, MA, USA) from the take-off line to the nearest point of landing contact (i.e., the back of the heels). Each athlete performed three jump attempts with 2 min intervals, and the longest distance was considered for further analysis.

3.2. Medicine Ball Throw Test

The procedures adopted for the medicine ball throw test assessment followed the protocol of Vossen et al. [19]. The warm-up and familiarization consisted of two–three submaximal throws prior to the test. The girls remained seated on the floor covered with judo mats and were stabilized with their backs supported against a vertical support, their thighs horizontally supported, their knees flexed at an angle of 90°, and their ankles resting on the floor. A 3 Kg medicine ball (Dynamax Inc®., Dallas, TX, USA) was positioned at the sternum of each athlete (point A), who then threw it with both hands without moving her trunk. When an athlete failed to maintain the established body orientation, the throw attempt was disregarded. The distance the medicine ball was thrown from point A up to its first contact with the floor (point B) was measured. Each participant performed three throws, with 2 min intervals, and the greatest distance achieved in the three attempts was considered for further analysis.

3.3. Handgrip Strength Test

Handgrip strength was measured using a handgrip dynamometer (Carci®, SH 5001 model), following the protocol used by Detanico et al. [8]. The warm-up and familiarization consisted of three rapid contractions performed during a 2 s period. The participants were instructed to sustain a maximal isometric contraction during each measurement (lasting

3 to 6 s). The three contractions were performed with the dominant (self-selected) hand with 2 min intervals, in the standing position with shoulder flexion at 90° and the elbow completely extended. The highest value obtained in the three trials was considered for further analysis.

3.4. Judo-Specific Tests

3.4.1. Special Judo Fitness Test

The SJFT is a judo high-intensity intermittent test developed by Sterkowicz [20]. The girls performed a 5 min warm-up before the test, which consisted of jogging, judo falling techniques (*ukemi*), and repetitive throwing techniques (*uchi-komi*). Subsequently, three athletes of similar body mass (with a maximum variation of 10%) and height performed the SJFT, according to the following protocol: two judokas were positioned at a distance of 6 m from each other, while the athlete being tested was positioned 3 m from the judokas to be thrown. The procedure was divided into three periods: 15 s (A), 30 s (B), and 30 s (C), with a 10 s interval between periods. In each period, the athlete being tested threw the other judoka using the one-arm shoulder throw (*ippon-seoi-nage*) technique as many times as possible. Performance was determined by the total throws completed during each of the three periods (SJFT$_{TT}$ = A + B + C). Heart rate (HR) was measured immediately after the test and then 1 min later by an HR monitor positioned on the chest (Polar® M430—Kempele/Finland). The SJFT$_{INDEX}$ was calculated as the change in heart rate (immediately after the test and 1 min later) divided by SJFT$_{TT}$. Previous study showed reliability values (Intraclass Correlation Coefficient—ICC) ranging from 0.71 to 0.81 for number of throws, heart rate (0.66–0.86), and SJFT index (0.87) [21].

3.4.2. Judogi Grip Strength Test

The girls were familiarized with the JGST by performing one sustained attempt of 2–3 s grasping a judo uniform (*judogi*) suspended on an elevated horizontal bar. The JGST consisted of sustaining a predefined position of elbow flexion for a maximum time. Athletes performed only the isometric version of the JGST (JGST$_{ISO}$). The chronometer began with a verbal command and was stopped when the participants could no longer maintain the original position. The reliability of the JGST has been assessed in a previous study, presenting an ICC higher than 0.98 [22].

4. Statistical Analysis

Data are reported as means and standard deviation (SD). The Shapiro–Wilk test was used to verify the normality of the data. Independent t-tests were used to compare the variables among girls at different menarcheal status. For the t-test, we used the Cohen's d, considering 0.0–0.2 as trivial, 0.21–0.6 as small, 0.61–1.2 as moderate, 1.21–2.0 as large, and 2.1–4.0 as very large [23]. Multiple linear regression analysis (backward stepwise method with criteria for entry of $p < 0.05$ and removal of $p < 0.10$) was used to estimate the relative contributions of age at menarche, chronological age, years of formal training, and growth measurements (height and body mass) to physical performance. All independent variables showed variance inflation factors <2, reflecting no multicollinearity, tolerance >0.1, showing acceptable multicollinearity, and absolute values of correlation coefficients <0.70 [24]. The level of significance was set at 5%, and the analyses were performed using the JASP software (version 0.11.1, University of Amsterdam, Amsterdam, The Netherlands).

5. Results

Table 1 shows the demographic characteristics, judo experience, body size, and physical performance of female judo athletes of different menarcheal status. It was verified that post-menarche girls were older, more experienced, taller, and heavier and presented higher performance in SJFT (throws and index) and SLJ than pre-menarche girls. The age at menarche ranged from 10 to 13 years.

Table 1. Mean ± SD of demographic characteristics, judo experience, body size, and physical performance in female judo athletes of different menarcheal status.

	Pre-Menarche (n = 7)	Post-Menarche (n = 12)	p	ES
Chronological age (years)	11.5 ± 0.9	15.4 ± 1.5	<0.01 *	2.98
Age at menarche (years)	–	11.8 ± 1.2	–	–
Training experience (years)	4.0 ± 2.2	6.4 ± 2.5	0.03 *	1.01
Body mass (kg)	45.3 ± 3.4	59.0 ± 11.3	<0.01 *	1.36
Height (cm)	150.8 ± 5.2	159.3 ± 6.2	<0.01 *	1.47
$SJFT_{TT}$ (n)	20 ± 1	23 ± 3	0.01 *	1.13
$SJFT_{HR\_FINAL}$ (bpm)	181 ± 4	183 ± 8	0.34	0.28
$SJFT_{HR\_1MIN}$ (bpm)	160 ± 6	154 ± 14	0.16	0.49
$SJFT_{INDEX}$	16.7 ± 1.1	14.9 ± 1.9	0.02 *	1.08
$JGST_{ISO}$ (s)	33.7 ± 9.8	43.9 ± 15.7	0.07	0.74
SLJ (cm)	177 ± 15	213 ± 45	0.04 *	0.90
MBT (cm)	277 ± 19	309 ± 71	0.15	0.50
HGS (kgf)	29.7 ± 6.9	34.8 ± 7.6	0.08	0.70

Note: * $p < 0.05$, SJFT: Special Judo Fitness Test, $SJFT_{TT}$: total throws of SJFT, $SJFT_{HR}$: heart rate during SJFT, $JGST_{ISO}$: Judogi Grip Strength Test, SLJ: Standing Long Jump Test, MBT: Medicine Ball Throw Test, HGS: Handgrip Strength Test.

Table 2 summarizes the indicators of the physical performance tests in post-menarcheal female judo athletes. The age at menarche and body mass (negative predictors) and the chronological age (positive predictor) explained 70% of the variance in $JGST_{ISO}$ performance. Judo training experience and chronological age (positive predictors) and age at menarche (negative predictor) explained 59% of the SLJ performance. Chronological age (positive predictor) and age at menarche (negative predictor) accounted for 40% of the variance in MBT performance, while chronological age and height (both positive predictors) explained 52% of the variance in HGS. For $SJFT_{TT}$, no predictive analysis was reported because no variable was entered in the model using the stepwise criteria.

Table 2. Indicators of the physical performance tests in young post-menarcheal female judo athletes.

	Adjusted R^2	p	Indicator	Standardized Coefficients (β)	p
$JGST_{ISO}$ (s)	0.70	<0.01	Age-menarche	−0.788	<0.01
			Chronological age	0.783	<0.01
			Body mass	−0.803	<0.01
SLJ (cm)	0.59	0.01	Training	0.476	0.05
			Chronological age	0.526	0.04
			Age-menarche	−0.382	0.10
MBT (cm)	0.40	0.04	Chronological age	0.731	0.01
			Age-menarche	−0.449	0.10
HGS (kgf)	0.52	0.01	Chronological age	0.585	0.02
			Height	0.446	0.06

Note: $JGST_{ISO}$: Judogi Grip Strength Test, SLJ: Standing Long Jump Test, MBT: Medicine Ball Throw Test, HGS: Handgrip Strength Test.

6. Discussion

The results of this study showed that post-menarche youth female judo athletes with advanced somatic growth presented higher performance in a judo-specific test (SJFT) and greater lower limb power output (SLJ) than their pre-menarche counterparts. Chronological age was an indicator in all physical tests, while age at menarche was an indicator for three of the four examined variables in post-menarche girls, thereby demonstrating that age-related maturity has an impact on general neuromuscular and judo-specific physical performance.

Similar to reports in team sports, post-menarcheal female judo athletes self-reported reaching their menarche close to 12 years. For example, Böhme [25] found the mean age at menarche to be close to 12.8 years in athletics, basketball, football, and handball athletes.

Menarcheal status is an indicator of sexual maturity and usually occurs from 11 to 15 years of age, following a growth spurt (i.e., PHV) [3,26] due to hormonal alterations [1,27]. From this developmental period, advancement of motor skills and physical performance is expected, especially if there is adequate involvement in physical and sports activities from an early age [28,29]. In this study, it was verified that post-menarche youth female athletes initiated practicing judo earlier than the pre-menarche group, which may be related to their higher physical performance.

It was also found that youth female judo athletes in the post-menarche group were older, taller, and heavier than those in the pre-menarche group. Generally, adolescent girls start their growth spurt quickly, increasing approximately 8–9 cm in height per year [1] and gaining approximately 2.3–2.7 kg of body mass annually [30]. Therefore, the higher chronological age and the advanced somatic growth processes (represented by body size measurements) of post-menarche girls may explain their higher physical performance, particularly, the number of throws in SJFT and SLJ performance. A previous study verified that the number of throws in the SJFT was positively correlated with vertical jump performance in adult male judo athletes [31]. Thus, higher levels of muscle power in the lower limbs of the post-menarche girls may help to explain their higher performance in SJFT. In addition, the greater time of formal training in post-menarche girls most likely contributed to increased muscle power, as Zaggelidis et al. [32] verified that judo training enhances vertical jump performance, mainly due to improvements in the stretch–shortening cycle (SSC).

Adolescent athletes with better aerobic function present higher performance in high-intensity intermittent efforts [33]. The ability of children to better maintain performance during repeated high-intensity exercise bouts could be related to a better optimization of oxidative pathways than of glycolytic pathways during exercise and to a lower activation of type II muscle fibers, resulting in greater resistance to fatigue [34]. Although aerobic fitness was not evaluated in this study, it is possible to suggest that post-menarche girls present a higher aerobic condition than pre-menarche girls, especially due to the previously reported correlation between SJFT performance and aerobic capacity [31]. In some neuromuscular tests (HGS, MBT, JGST), there were no significant differences between pre- and post-menarche girls.

When specific indicators of physical tests were investigated in post-menarche youth judo athletes, the age at menarche was found to be negatively associated with $JGST_{ISO}$, SLJ, and MBT (i.e., the earlier the age at menarche, the higher the performance). The status of menarche represents a great gain in the release of progesterone, estrogen, and, to a lesser extent, testosterone [35,36]. The release of estrogen and testosterone is linked to increased muscle mass and body fat, which have positive and negative influences on physical performance, respectively. In addition, the release of these hormones has been related to increases in lactic anaerobic power [37] and maximum aerobic power due to the growth of body dimensions [38].

Chronological age was a positive indicator of all neuromuscular tests, potentially demonstrating a major influence on physical performance tests in post-menarche youth female judo athletes. Detanico et al. [8] previously verified that chronological age was a positive indicator of judo-specific performance ($JGST_{ISO}$ and SJFT variables) in young male judo athletes. Similarly, a study conducted by Courel-Ibanez et al. [39] detected a higher number of throws in the SJFT in U15 male amateur judo athletes compared to U13 athletes, showing better performance in older boys, especially when utilizing anaerobic pathways. Giudicelli et al. [12] also found that older male judokas (aged 11.0–14.7 years) performed better in most of the physical tests; however, in their study, the maturation attenuated the age effect in most variables and significantly affected upper body strength.

Another interesting finding was that the number of years of formal training was positively associated with SLJ performance, showing improvements in muscle power of the lower limbs in post-menarche girls with judo training experience. A previous investigation found that vertical jump performance discriminated adult judo athletes with different training experience levels (advanced vs. novice) [40], likely due to SSC enhancements [32]. Moreover, muscle power of the lower limbs is an important parameter related to technical–tactical performance during judo matches in senior female athletes [41].

Somatic growth variables (height and body mass) were positive and negative indicators of HGS and $JGST_{ISO}$, respectively. Taller girls obtained advantages in the HGS test, probably due to the longer forearm and arm [1,42], which may be related to increased force production capacity. This finding exhibits practical relevance, since gripping tasks are an important component of judo performance [43]. Concurrently, body mass showed a negative impact on $JGST_{ISO}$ performance. This test estimates isometric endurance strength in the upper body [22], and to perform it, the athletes must hold onto a bar and suspend themselves (i.e., hold their own body mass). The JGST has been previously shown to have a negative relationship with body mass [44], suggesting that heavier athletes may underperform in absolute terms in this specific test.

Finally, some limitations of this study should be addressed, such as the small sample size, particularly after division into groups according to the menarcheal status. However, the statistical power calculated a posteriori presented values >0.8 for the variables that showed significant differences, thus avoiding type II error. Nonetheless, this is the first investigation examining the effects of menarcheal status and growth on physical performance in young female judo athletes. The current results expose differences in physical performance according to the menarcheal status, showing that post-menarche girls are stronger and perform better than pre-menarche counterparts. This highlights the importance of having pre-menarche girls compete in their own age category and not in higher age groups. Age at menarche, chronological age, growth, and years of formal judo training seemed to explain the performance in post-menarche female athletes. These indicators seem to contribute to competitive success, as it was found that years of formal training, height, and strength tests performance ($JGST_{ISO}$ and SLJ) can discriminate the competitive level in young male judo athletes (national vs. state level) [9]. However, to prevent exposure to early specialization, it is essential to consider the maturation characteristics of female youth judo athletes and individualize training loads during short- and medium-term planning. These actions will contribute to avoid harmful effects of early specialization on physical and mental health during childhood and adolescence. We recommend for future studies to investigate the influence of ethnicity, population size, parents' education, socio-economic and nutritional parameters, as it is known that age at menarche is a sensitive indicator of environmental conditions during childhood.

7. Conclusions

We concluded that post-menarcheal youth female judo athletes are older, more advanced in the growth process, more experienced in judo, and present higher physical performance when compared to girls who have not yet reached menarche. Chronological age and the age at menarche were shown to be the greatest indicators of neuromuscular and judo-specific performance in post-menarche youth female judo athletes. Furthermore, somatic growth and years of formal training also contributed to neuromuscular performance of the upper and lower limbs.

Author Contributions: Conceptualization, M.S.d.S.A., R.L.K. and D.D.; Methodology, M.S.d.S.A., R.L.K. and D.D.; Formal analysis, M.S.d.S.A., R.L.K. and D.D.; Investigation, M.S.d.S.A., R.L.K., D.H.F. and D.D.; Data curation, M.S.d.S.A. and R.L.K.; Writing original draft preparation, M.S.d.S.A., R.L.K., D.H.F. and D.D.; Visualization, M.S.d.S.A., R.L.K., D.H.F. and D.D.; Supervision, D.D. and D.H.F.; Project administration, D.D. All authors have read and agreed to the published version of the manuscript.

Funding: This work was financed by The Coordination for the Improvement of Higher Education Personnel (CAPES)—PROEX n°: 23038.007266/2021-94.

Institutional Review Board Statement: The study was conducted according to the guidelines of the Declaration of Helsinki and approved by the Research Ethics Committee of the local university (Federal University of Santa Catarina, number: 63053516.4.0000.0121).

Informed Consent Statement: Informed consent was obtained from all subjects involved in the study.

Data Availability Statement: The data are not publicly available for ethical privacy reasons with the subjects involved in the research.

Conflicts of Interest: The authors declare no conflict of interest.

References

1. Malina, R.M.; Bouchard, C.; Bar-Or, O. *Growth, Maturation, and Physical Activity*, 2nd ed.; Human Kinetics: Champaign, IL, USA, 2004.
2. Mirwald, R.L.; Baxter-Jones, A.D.G.; Bailey, D.A.; Beunen, G.P. An assessment of maturity from anthropometric measurements. *Med. Sci. Sports Exerc.* **2002**, *34*, 689–694.
3. Malina, R.M.; Rogol, A.D.; Cumming, S.P.; e Coelho Silva, M.J.; Figueiredo, A.J. Biological maturation of youth athletes: Assessmentand implications. *Br. J. Sports Med.* **2015**, *49*, 852–859. [CrossRef]
4. Carvalho, H.M.; Gonçalves, C.E.; Grosgeorge, B.; Paes, R.R. Validity and usefulness of the Line Drill test for adolescent basketball players: A Bayesian multilevel analysis. *Res. Sports Med.* **2017**, *25*, 333–344. [CrossRef]
5. Coelho, E.; Silva, M.J.; Figueiredo, A.J.; Simões, F.; Seabra, A.; Natal, A.; Vaeyens, R.; Philippaerts, R.; Cumming, S.P.; Malina, R.M. Discrimination of u-14 soccer players by level and position. *Int. J. Sport Med.* **2010**, *31*, 790–796. [CrossRef] [PubMed]
6. Figueiredo, A.J.; Gonçalves, C.E.; Coelho e Silva, M.J.; Malina, R.M. Youth soccer players, 11-14 years: Maturity, size, function, skill and goal orientation. *Ann. Hum. Biol.* **2009**, *36*, 60–73. [CrossRef] [PubMed]
7. Teixeira, A.S.; Guglielmo, L.G.A.; Fernandes-da-Silva, J.; Konarski, J.M.; Costa, D.; Duarte, J.P.; Malina, R.M. Skeletal maturity and oxygen uptake in youth soccer controlling for concurrent size descriptors. *PLoS ONE* **2018**, *13*, e0205976. [CrossRef] [PubMed]
8. Detanico, D.; Kons, R.L.; Fukuda, D.H.; Teixeira, A.S. Physical Performance in Young Judo Athletes: Influence of Somatic Maturation, Growth and Training Experience. *Res. Q. Exerc. Sport* **2020**, *91*, 425–432. [CrossRef]
9. Detanico, D.; Kons, R.L.; Canestri, R.; Albuquerque, M. Can judo experience, somatic maturation, growth and physical capacities discriminate young judo athletes from different competitive levels? *High Abil. Stud.* **2021**, ahead of print. [CrossRef]
10. Fukuda, D.H.; Beyer, K.S.; Boone, C.H.; Wang, R.; La Monica, M.B.; Wells, A.J.; Hoffman, J.R.; Jeffrey, R.; Stout, J.R. Developmental associations with muscle morphology, physical performance, and asymmetry in youth judo athletes. *Sport Sci. Health* **2018**, *14*, 555–562. [CrossRef]
11. Giudicelli, B.B.; Luz, L.G.O.; Sogut, M.; Massart, A.G.; Júnior, A.C.; António, J.; Figueiredo, A.J. Bio-Banding in Judo: The Mediation Role of Anthropometric Variables on the Maturation Effect. *Int. J. Environ. Res. Public Health* **2020**, *17*, 361. [CrossRef]
12. Giudicelli, B.B.; Luz, L.G.O.; Sogut, M.; Sarmento, H.; Massart, A.G.; Júnior, A.C.; Field, A.; Figueiredo, A.J. Chronological Age, Somatic Maturation and Anthropometric Measures: Association with Physical Performance of Young Male Judo Athletes. *Int. J. Environ. Res. Public Health* **2021**, *18*, 6410. [CrossRef]
13. Franchini, E.; Del Vecchio, F.B.; Matsushigue, K.A.; Artioli, G.G. Physiological profiles of elite judo athletes. *Sports Med.* **2011**, *41*, 147–166. [CrossRef] [PubMed]
14. IJF—International Judo Federation. Rules. Home Page. Available online: https://www.ijf.org/ (accessed on 1 August 2021).
15. Sherar, L.B.; Baxter-Jones, A.D.G.; Mirwald, R.L. Limitations to the use of secondary sex characteristics for gender comparisons. *Ann. Hum. Biol.* **2004**, *31*, 586–593. [CrossRef] [PubMed]
16. Leonardi, T.J.; Paes, R.R.; Breder, L.; Foster, C.; Gonçalves, C.E.; Carvalho, H.M. Biological maturation, training experience, body size and functional capacity of adolescent female basketball players: A Bayesian analysis. *Int. J. Sports Sci. Coach* **2018**, *13*, 713–722. [CrossRef]
17. Camargo, C.T.A.; Gomez-Campos, R.A.; Cossio-Bolaños, M.A.; Barbeta, V.J.O.; Arruda, M.; Guerra-Junior, G. Growth and body composition in Brazilian female rhythmic gymnastics athletes. *J. Sports Sci.* **2014**, *32*, 1790–1796. [CrossRef] [PubMed]
18. Pinto, V.C.M.; Santos, P.G.M.D.; Medeiros, R.S.C.S.; Souza, F.E.S.; Simões, T.B.S.; de Carvalho Dantas, R.P.N.; Cabral, B.G.D.A.T. Maturational stages: Comparison of growth and physical capacity indicators in adolescents. *J. Hum. Growth Dev.* **2018**, *28*, 42–49. [CrossRef]
19. Vossen, J.F.; Kramerdarren, J.E.; Burke, D.G.; Vossen, D.P. Comparison of dynamic push-up training and plyometric push-up training on upper-body power and strength. *J. Strength Cond. Res.* **2000**, *14*, 248–253.
20. Sterkowicz, S. Test Specjalnej Sprawno ś ci Ruchowej w Judo. *Antropomotoryka* **1995**, *12*, 29–44.
21. Štefanovský, M.; Poliak, M.; Augustovičová, D.; Kraček, S.; Hadža, R. Test and Re-Test Reliability of the Special Judo Fitness Test. *Acta Fac. Educ. Phys. Univ. Comen.* **2021**, *61*, 97–106. [CrossRef]
22. Franchini, E.; Miarka, B.; Matheus, L.; Del Vecchio, F.B. Endurance in judogi grip strength tests: Comparison between elite and non-elite judo players. *Arch. Budo* **2011**, *7*, 1–4.
23. Cohen, J. *Statistical Power for the Social Sciences*; Laurence Erlbaum Assoc.: Hillsdale, NJ, USA, 1988.

24. Dormann, C.F.; Elith, J.; Bacher, S.; Buchmann, C.; Carl, G.; Carré, G.; Marquéz, J.R.G.; Gruber, B.; Lafourcade, B.; Leitão, P.J.; et al. Collinearity: A review of methods to deal with it and a simulation study evaluating their performance. *Ecography* **2012**, *35*, 1–20. [CrossRef]
25. Böhme, M.T.S. Aerobic endurance in young female athletes in respect to sexual maturation, age and growth. *Rev. Bras. Cineantropometria Desempenho Hum.* **2004**, *6*, 27–35. (In Portuguese)
26. McManus, A.M.; Armstrong, N. Physiology of elite young female athletes. *Med. Sport Sci.* **2011**, *56*, 23–46. [PubMed]
27. Rogol, A.D.; Roemmich, J.N.; Clark, P.A. Growth at puberty. *J. Adolesc. Health* **2002**, *31*, 192–200. [CrossRef]
28. Jones, M.A.; Hitchen, P.J.; Stratton, G. The importance of considering biological maturity when assessing physical fitness measures in girls and boys aged 10 to 16 years. *Ann. Hum. Biol.* **2000**, *27*, 57–65. [CrossRef]
29. Volver, A.; Viru, A.; Viru, M. Improvement of motor abilities in pubertal girls. *J. Sports Med. Phys. Fit.* **2000**, *40*, 17–25. [PubMed]
30. Sinclair, D.; Dangerfield, P. *Human Growth after Birth*, 6th ed.; Oxford University Press: New York, NY, USA, 1998.
31. Detanico, D.; Dal Pupo, J.; Franchini, E.; Santos, S.G. Relationship of aerobic and neuromuscular indexes with specific actions in judo. *Sci. Sports* **2012**, *27*, 16–22. [CrossRef]
32. Zaggelidis, G.; Lazaridis, S.N.; Malkogiorgos, A.; Mavrovouniotis, F. Differences in vertical jumping performance between untrained males and advanced Greek judokas. *Arch. Budo* **2012**, *8*, 87–90. [CrossRef]
33. Doncaster, G.; Marwood, S.; Iga, J.; Unnithan, V. Influence of oxygen uptake kinetics on physical performance in youth soccer. *Eur. J. Appl. Physiol.* **2016**, *116*, 1781–1794. [CrossRef] [PubMed]
34. Ratel, S.; Duché, P.; Williams, C.A. Muscle fatigue during high-intensity exercise in children. *Sports Med.* **2006**, *36*, 1031–1065. [CrossRef]
35. Lowe, D.A.; Baltgalvis, K.A.; Greising, S.M. Mechanisms behind estrogen's beneficial effect on muscle strength in females. *Exerc. Sport Sci. Rev.* **2010**, *38*, 61–67. [CrossRef]
36. Sarwar, R.; Niclos, B.B.; Rutherford, O.M. Changes in muscle strength, relaxation rate and fatiguability during the human menstrual cycle. *J. Physiol.* **1996**, *5*, 267–272. [CrossRef] [PubMed]
37. Lee, E.C.; Fragala, M.S.; Kavouras, S.A.; Queen, R.M.; Pryor, J.K.; Casa, D.J. Biomarkers in Sports and Exercise: Tracking Health, Performance, and Recovery in Athletes. *J. Strength Cond. Res.* **2017**, *31*, 2920–2937. [CrossRef]
38. Inbar, O.; Bar-Or, O. Anaerobic characteristics in male children and adolescents. *Med. Sci. Sports Exerc.* **1986**, *18*, 264–269. [CrossRef] [PubMed]
39. Courel-Ibáñez, J.; Franchini, E.; Escobar-Molina, R. Is the Special Judo Fitness Test Index discriminative during formative stages? Age and competitive level differences in U13 and U15 children. *Ido Mov. Cult. J. Martial Arts Anthropol.* **2018**, *18*, 37–41.
40. Detanico, D.; Dal Pupo, J.; Graup, S.; Santos, S.G. Vertical jump performance and isokinetic torque discriminate advanced and novice judo athletes. *Kinesiology* **2016**, *48*, 103–108. [CrossRef]
41. Kons, R.L.; Dal Pupo, J.; Ache-Dias, J.; Detanico, D. Female Judo Athletes' Physical Test Performances Are Unrelated to Technical-Tactical Competition Skills. *Percept. Mot. Skills* **2018**, *125*, 802–816. [CrossRef]
42. Yabanci, N.; Kiliç, S.; Simşek, I. The relationship between height and arm span, mid-upper arm and waist circumferences in children. *Ann. Hum.* **2010**, *37*, 70–75. [CrossRef]
43. Calmet, M.; Miarka, B.; Franchini, E. Modeling of grasps in judo contests. *Int. J. Perform. Anal. Sport* **2010**, *10*, 229–240. [CrossRef]
44. Branco, B.H.M.; Diniz, E.; Da Silva Santos, J.F.; Shiroma, S.A.; Franchini, E. Normative tables for the dynamic and isometric judogi chin-up tests for judo athletes. *Sport Sci. Health* **2016**, *13*, 47–53. [CrossRef]

Article

Analysis of Anthropometric and Body Composition Profile in Male and Female Traditional Rowers

Alfonso Penichet-Tomas, Basilio Pueo *, Sergio Selles-Perez and Jose M. Jimenez-Olmedo

Physical Education and Sports, Faculty of Education, University of Alicante, 03690 Alicante, Spain; alfonso.penichet@ua.es (A.P.-T.); sergio.selles@ua.es (S.S.-P.); j.olmedo@ua.es (J.M.J.-O.)
* Correspondence: basilio@ua.es

Abstract: The anthropometric profile has a fundamental role in rowing performance and young talent detection. The objective of this study was to analyze the anthropometric profile, body composition, and somatotype in traditional rowers, and to analyze which variables can be used as predictors of rowing performance. Twenty-four rowers competing at national level participated in this study, thirteen men and eleven women. Significant differences ($p < 0.001$) were observed in the height of male rowers (large effect size, $d = 1.8$) and in body mass (very large effect size, $d = 2.4$). Also, muscle mass reached a higher percentage in male rowers ($d = 3.7$), whereas the sum of seven skinfolds ($d = 2.0$) and body fat percentage ($d = 2.0$) reached higher values in female rowers, all their difference being significant ($p < 0.001$) with very large effect size. The somatotype of male rowers was ecto-mesomorph (1.8-4.5-3.0), and the somatotype of female rowers was in the balanced mesomorph (2.8-3.8-2.6). A very strong correlation between height ($r = 0.75$; $p = 0.002$) and rowing performance was found in male rowers. Body mass ($r = 0.70$; $p = 0.009$) and muscle mass ($r = 0.83$; $p = 0.001$) showed also very strong correlation in female rowers. Finally, height was the best predictor of performance for male rowers ($R^2 = 0.56$, $p < 0.003$) and muscle mass for female rowers ($R^2 = 0.68$, $p < 0.002$). The anthropometric profile of male and female traditional rowers showed differences to be considered in training programs and talent selection.

Keywords: rowing; anthropometry; somatotype; performance; talent identification

1. Introduction

Rowing is a sport that consists of propelling a boat through the water using one or more oars. The difference with other sports that also use oars is that the oars are fixed to the body of the boat with the rower positioned towards the bow of the boat resulting in the production of different dynamic force components [1,2]. The main classification of rowing modalities differentiates between boats with a mobile seat or a fixed seat [3].

The modality with mobile seat boats is generally called Olympic rowing because only this modality includes Olympic boats. The seat of each rower is placed on rails that allow forward and backward movement. The legs produce almost half the power of the drive (46%) while the trunk around 32% and the arms 22% [4]. The competitions, which can last between 5 and 8 min depending on the type of boat and the category, are generally over the distance of 2000 m in calm waters [5]. On the other hand, in fixed seat boats, the seats do not move in the boat and the technical execution is different since the rowers are supported in the coccyx area. This technical difference that prevents the rower from using the legs in such a wide range of motion implies that the amplitude of the trunk degree is greater than in Olympic rowing [6]. This modality is also called traditional rowing because it is how rowing was originally practiced: Llaüt, with eight rowers and a coxswain [7], and Trainera, with 13 rowers and a coxswain [8]. In addition, traditional rowing courses are not held in parallel lanes, but between two and four lengths with one or three complete tacks, both in calm water and the sea. These technical and competitive differences between modalities, boats, and types of competition result in different functional and physiological demands [9], where anthropometric characteristics and body composition have a fundamental role in Olympic [10,11] and traditional [7,12] rowing performance.

Most studies about anthropometry, body composition, and somatotype have focused on Olympic rowing [13–17]. Furthermore, some studies have not only compared the different profiles based on weight or age category. The differences between male and female rowers have also been analyzed, finding differences and similarities in anthropometric characteristics that could determine not only training programs but also offering indicators to be able to perform talent detection programs [18–20]. Even De Larochelambert [10] determined which morphologies (tall and thin, tall and robust, small and thin, or small and robust) had a significant effect on speed for both male and female rowers. On the other hand, the research also seem to determine that there are anthropometric characteristics that are related to the level of rowing performance such as height and length measurements [21]. Taller rowers can perform a wider stroke in the water, and a greater stroke range is directly related to increased rowing performance [22]. A similar trend is found with the body mass of the rowers since higher values seem to be correlated with success in competition [14]. Higher body mass can be a disadvantage for performance in other sports where the athlete must shift their own weight. In rowing, the rower is sitting in the boat and his own weight does not seem to have a negative effect on performance. These characteristics are above all in the heavyweight categories because in the lightweight categories the differences and correlations with success in rowing are lower [20]. The studies carried out show that in the heavyweight categories the body mass does not have a negative impact, even a greater weight positively favors power production. However, in the lightweight categories this fact has not been demonstrated as strongly. The profitability of the rower may have a greater impact. Nevertheless, a higher percentage of body fat can be a disadvantage [18]. The body composition of rowers is characterized by a low percentage of fat mass and a mesomorph body type associated with a high development of muscle mass as somatotype [15,16]. It has been widely reported that anthropometric variables and success in rowing are associated, which shows that these characteristics could be used as predictors of performance [23]. Even carrying out a complete body composition study with quantitative and qualitative parameters can be used to plan specific training cycles in different periods of the season [24].

Research in traditional rowing about anthropometry and body composition profile is very limited. Some researchers have studied the relationship of anthropometric characteristics with traditional rowing performance and some of these findings seem to coincide with the Olympic rowing modality, such as a greater body mass and fat-free mass seem to have a positive impact on rowing performance [12]. However, there are some differences such as less muscle mass [25] or lower average height that seem not as important to performance in traditional rowers [8]. Traditional rowing boats require rowers of different heights and weights for hydrodynamic reasons to balance the boat in rough seas [8]. For example, Sebastia-Amat et al. [26] found that only body mass for male rowers and body muscle for female rowers were good predictors of performance in traditional rowing.

Further investigation of these differences between modalities and gender is essential to determine a complete profile of the traditional rower and for following objective criteria in talent recruitment programs. Furthermore, changes in some characteristics of body composition in rowers can be a performance advantage, so control and monitoring of body composition can be crucial for their success in competition [24]. For this reason and because there is also no scientific evidence of comparative studies that carry out a complete study of body composition profile of traditional rowers, the objective of this study is to analyze and compare the anthropometric profile, body composition, and somatotype in male and female traditional rowers. In addition, the present study also aims to analyze the anthropometric variables that influence rowing performance and which of them can be used as predictors of performance. Despite general variations between genders are expected, the differences will allow to create a differentiated profile of rowers competing at the national level and to verify that characteristics such as height and weight, among others, have a relevant role in rowing performance.

2. Materials and Methods

2.1. Participants

Twenty-four rowers competing at national level participated in this study, thirteen males (age: 27.3 ± 5.1 years; height: 182.1 ± 6.6 cm, body mass: 75.3 ± 5.3 kg) and eleven females (age: 27.7 ± 4.3 years; height: 169.9 ± 6.7 cm, body mass: 61.9 ± 6.0 kg). The requirement to participate was to have qualified for the national championship, with an experience of at least 3 years, and to regularly train a minimum of six days per week for 2–3 h/day, supervised by one of the authors who perform the physical preparation and monitoring of the athletes who have participated in the study. They were asked to refrain from eating for at least four hours before the measurements, not exercise on the day of the measurement [16] and not high intensity exercise the day before. The hydration guidelines were the same as those carried out for training, no specific hydration guidelines were given. All measurements were made at the same time of the day. Rowers who did not meet the selection criteria were excluded from the study. The Ethics Committee of the University of Alicante gave institutional approval for this study, in accordance with the Declaration of Helsinki (IRB UA-2020-07-21). The subjects were informed about the study and gave their written informed consent.

2.2. Procedure

The anthropometric assessment followed the guidelines set by the International Society for the Advancement of Kinanthropometry (ISAK) [27]. The measurements were performed by the same researcher with ISAK certification level II under fasting conditions at room temperature (22 ± 1 °C) [28,29]. All variables were measured on the right side of the body in duplicate and the mean value was recorded. Intra-observer technical error of the measurement (TEM), 5% for skinfolds and 1% for girths and breadths, was considered for the measurements.

Body mass and height were measured using a scale (model 707, Seca, Hamburg, Germany) to the nearest 0.1 kg and a stadiometer (Harpenden, Burgess Hill, UK) to the nearest 0.1 cm. Rowers were weighted and measured wearing only underwear with bare feet. Height was measured with the rower completely upright and the chin parallel with the ground. Body mass index (BMI) was computed as body mass (kg) divided by height squared (m^2). Eight skinfolds (triceps, biceps, subscapular, iliac crest, supraspinal, abdominal, front thigh, and calf) were measured with a Holtain skinfold caliper to the nearest 0.2 mm and six girths (relaxed arm, tensed arm, thigh, medial calf, waist, and hip) were obtained using a Holtain bone breadth caliper to the nearest 0.1 cm (Holtain Ltd., Crymych, UK). The sum of eight skinfolds was examined following validated procedures [30]. Finally, three breadths (humerus, femur, and stylion) were measured with an anthropometric tape (Seca) to the nearest 0.1 cm. Fat, muscle, bone, and residual masses were calculated, as well as somatotype. To calculate the percentage of body fat, the formula of Withers et al. was used [30]. Muscle mass was determined using the methods of Lee et al. [31] and bone mass was calculated following the Rocha model [32]. The anthropometric somatotype was determined using the Carter and Heath equation [33], making a graphic representation of the results in a somatochart.

Once the anthropometric study was completed, the rowers performed an all-out 2000 m test on a rowing ergometer (Model D; Concept 2, Inc., Morrisville, VT, USA) with a coupling adapted for the reproduction of the traditional rowing stroke fixing the seat [25,34] and with a PM5 performance monitor to collect mean power output reached in the test, and its equivalence in time. All the rowers were familiar with the rowing machine and with the drag factor used: 160 for males and 140 for females. The rowers performed a 10-min warm-up before the test at moderate intensity between 70 to 80% of maximum heart rate (above 140 beats per min) at a stroke rate of 18–20 strokes per minute [26]. Power output, stroke rate and time to complete 2000 m rowing ergometer performance test were recorded.

2.3. Statistical Analysis

Descriptive analysis was presented by the mean, standard deviation (SD), minimum (min), and maximum (max) for all variables. Shapiro–Wilk statistical test was used to verify that the variables followed the normality criterion. Student's t-test was used to compare anthropometric data between male and female rowers. Cohen's d was used as a measure of the effect size of differences between male and female rowers and interpreted according to modified thresholds [35] for sports sciences [36] as trivial (<0.2), small (0.21–0.6), moderate (0.61–1.2), large (1.2–1.99), and very large (>2.0). Somatotype Attitudinal Mean (SAM) and Somatotype Attitudinal Variance (SAV) were calculated to describe the magnitude of the dispersion of somatotypes in both groups. Somatotype Attitudinal Distance (SAD), the distance in three dimensions between male and female groups, was used to compare somatotype group means. Pearson correlation coefficient (r) was used to determine relationships between each anthropometric variable with rowing performance. Effect sizes of relationships were assessed by Pearson's correlations and coefficients of determination: trivial (<0.1), small (0.1–0.29), moderate (0.3–0.49), strong (0.5–0.69), very strong (0.7–0.89), nearly perfect (0.9–0.99), and perfect (1.0) [36]. A stepwise multiple regression analysis ($R^2 > 0.5$) was used to analyze which anthropometric variables could be used to predict rowing performances. Statistical significance was set at $p < 0.05$. Statistical analyses were performed using Statistical Package for Social Sciences (SPSS v.26 for Windows, SPSS Inc., Chicago, IL, USA).

3. Results

Body mass, height, and BMI mean values were significantly higher ($p < 0.05$) in male rowers (182.1 ± 6.6 cm, 75.3 ± 5.3 kg, and 22.8 ± 1.3 kg/m^2) than female rowers (169.9 ± 6.7 cm, body mass: 61.9 ± 6.0 kg 21.4 ± 1.0 kg/m^2) with large to very large effect size, as shown in Table 1. However, the skinfolds of triceps, biceps, iliac crest, front thigh, and calf were significantly higher ($p < 0.05$) in female rowers than in male rowers, with moderate to very large effect size. Therefore, the mean of the sum of skinfolds also showed a larger value in female rowers (88.0 ± 17.6 mm) than in male rowers (58.5 ± 12.4 mm). This difference was statistically significant ($p < 0.001$) with very large effect size ($d = 2.0$). In contrast, most of the girths were significantly higher ($p < 0.05$) in male rowers than in female rowers, with moderate effect size on thigh girth ($d = 0.9$) and very large effect size on relaxed arm ($d = 2.5$), tensed arm ($d = 3.4$) and waist girths ($d = 2.7$). Finally, humerus ($d = 2.7$), femur ($d = 1.8$) and stylion breadths ($d = 3.0$) also reached statistically higher values in male rowers, with large to very large effect size.

Table 2 shows body composition and somatotype profile of male and female rowers which highlights that male rower reached larger values of muscle mass (46.7 ± 2.0%) than female rowers (39.1 ± 2.1%), with significant difference ($p < 0.001$; $d = 3.7$) and very large effect size. However, female rowers achieved higher fat (15.4 ± 3.1%) and residual masses (29.4 ± 1.9%) than male rowers (10.3 ± 2.1% and 26.4 ± 1.9%, respectively). This contrast showed significant differences ($p < 0.001$) and very large ($d = 2.0$) and large ($d = 1.6$) effect size, respectively.

The comparative analysis of the somatotype between male and female rowers indicates that there are significant differences in endomorphy ($p < 0.001$; $d = 2.0$), with very large effect size, and mesomorphy ($p < 0.001$; $d = 1.8$), with large effect size. The mean somatotype of male rowers was mesomorph-ectomorph (1.8-4.5-3.8) and the mean somatotype of female rowers was balanced mesomorph (2.9-3.0-2.9) (Figure 1). Finally, SAM values were 1.1 in male rowers and 0.9 in female rowers where no significant differences between them, and the effect size was small ($d = 0.2$). The difference in SAD between male and female rowers was 1.0.

Table 1. Mean values of anthropometric measurements and difference between male and female rowers.

	Male (n = 13)		Female (n = 11)		t-Test		Cohen's d	
	Mean ± SD	Min–Max	Mean ± SD	Min–Max	p	95% CI	d	Effect Size
Basic measurements								
Age (years)	27.3 ± 5.1	20.0–37.0	27.7 ± 4.3	21.0–35.0	0.831	−4.5–3.6	0.08	Trivial
Body mass (kg)	75.3 ± 5.3 *	66.0–83.1	61.9 ± 6.0	51.8–69.6	<0.001	8.7–18.2	2.4	Very large
Height (cm)	182.1 ± 6.6 *	174.0–193.0	169.9 ± 6.7	160.0–178.0	<0.001	6.5–17.8	1.8	Large
BMI (kg/m^2)	22.8 ± 1.3 *	20.8–24.5	21.4 ± 1.0	20.1–23.6	0.010	0.4–2.3	1.2	Large
Skinfolds								
Triceps (mm)	6.2 ± 1.7	3.0–10.0	12.1 ± 2.4 *	7.0–15.0	<0.001	−7.6–−4.1	2.9	Very large
Biceps (mm)	2.7 ± 0.7	2.0–4.0	4.4 ± 1.4 *	2.0–6.0	0.004	−2.7–−0.6	1.6	Large
Subscapular (mm)	7.7 ± 1.4	6.0–10.0	8.1 ± 1.8	6.0–11.0	0.463	−1.9–0.9	0.3	Small
Iliac crest (mm)	9.7 ± 3.4	5.0–15.0	13.4 ± 3.8 *	9.0–21.0	0.020	−6.7–−0.6	1.0	Moderate
Supraspinal (mm)	6.8 ± 1.9	4.0–10.0	8.5 ± 2.7	6.0–13.0	0.088	−3.7–0.3	0.8	Moderate
Abdominal (mm)	10.2 ± 3.4	6.0–16.0	12.1 ± 4.5	6.0–20.0	0.222	−5.4–1.3	0.5	Small
Front thigh (mm)	10.1 ± 2.9	6.0–15.0	18.4 ± 4.5 *	11.0–24.0	<0.001	−11.4–−5.1	3.5	Very large
Calf (mm)	5.1 ± 1.7	3.0–9.0	10.9 ± 3.6 *	6.0–18.0	<0.001	−8.3–−3.3	2.0	Very large
Σ 8 skinfolds (mm)	58.5 ± 12.4	37.0–75.0	88.0 ± 17.6 *	61.0–117.0	<0.001	−42.1–−16.9	2.0	Very large
Girths								
Relaxed arm (cm)	31.0 ± 2.0 *	27.5–34.0	26.5 ± 1.5	24.0–29.0	<0.001	3.0–6.0	2.5	Very large
Tensed arm (cm)	34.6 ± 2.1 *	30.5–37.5	28.6 ± 1.2	27.0–30.8	<0.001	4.5–7.4	3.4	Very large
Thigh (cm)	54.1 ± 2.2 *	48.5–56.5	52.1 ± 2.3	48.0–56.0	0.034	0.2–4.0	0.9	Moderate
Medial calf (cm)	37.2 ± 3.3	27.0–39.5	36.0 ± 1.9	33.0–39.5	0.297	−1.1–3.5	0.4	Small
Waist (cm)	79.6 ± 3.0 *	74.5–85.0	70.5 ± 3.9	65.0–76.0	<0.001	6.2–12.1	2.7	Very large
Hip (cm)	95.3 ± 3.4	88.0–99.0	95.9 ± 4.9	89.5–106.0	0.763	−4.0–3.0	0.1	Trivial
Breadths								
Humerus (cm)	7.1 ± 0.3 *	6.5–7.5	6.3 ± 0.3	5.7–6.6	<0.001	0.6–1.1	2.7	Very large
Femur (cm)	9.7 ± 0.4 *	9.0–10.0	9.0 ± 0.4	8.5–9.5	<0.001	0.3–1.0	1.8	Large
Stylion (cm)	5.7 ± 0.2 *	5.4–6.5	5.1 ± 0.2	4.7–5.5	<0.001	0.4–0.9	3.0	Very large

BMI: Body Mass Index; SD: standard deviation; min: minimum; max: maximum; CI: confidence interval; *: statistically significance between male and female rowers ($p < 0.05$).

Table 2. Descriptive data and comparative analysis of body composition and somatotype between male and female rowers.

	Male (n = 13)		Female (n = 11)		t-Test		Cohen's d	
	Mean ± SD	Min–Max	Mean ± SD	Min–Max	p	95% CI	d	Effect Size
Body composition								
Fat mass (%)	10.3 ± 2.1	6.6–13.1	15.4 ± 3.1 *	10.7–20.5	<0.001	−7.3–−3.0	2.0	Very large
Muscle mass (%)	46.7 ± 2.0 *	43.1–49.7	39.1 ± 2.1	35.2–43.5	<0.001	5.8–9.3	3.7	Very large
Bone mass (%)	16.2 ± 2.2	10.1–18.6	16.0 ± 0.8	14.7–17.4	0.754	−1.2–1.6	0.1	Trivial
Residual mass (%)	26.4 ± 1.9	22.9–29.0	29.4 ± 1.9 *	26.2–32.5	<0.001	−4.6–−1.4	1.6	Large
Fat mass (kg)	7.8 ± 1.9	4.38–10.4	9.6 ± 2.4	5.7–12.9	0.051	−3.6–0.1	0.8	Moderate
Muscle mass (kg)	35.1 ± 2.3 *	31.9–38.6	24.2 ± 2.4	20.4–28.0	<0.001	8.9–12.9	4.7	Very large
Bone mass (kg)	12.5 ± 1.2 *	11.1–15.4	9.9 ± 1.0	8.4–11.2	<0.001	1.7–3.5	2.3	Very large
Residual mass (kg)	19.9 ± 1.9 *	16.7–22.6	18.2 ± 1.9	14.7–20.1	0.039	0.1–3.3	0.9	Moderate
Somatotype								
Endomorphy	1.8 ± 0.5	1.0–2.4	2.9 ± 0.6 *	2.1–4.0	<0.001	−1.5–−0.6	2.0	Very large
Mesomorphy	4.5 ± 0.9 *	3.1–6.5	3.0 ± 0.7	1.7–4.0	<0.001	0.9–2.2	1.8	Large
Ectomorphy	3.0 ± 0.8	1.8–3.9	2.9 ± 0.6	1.5–3.5	0.685	−0.5–0.7	0.1	Trivial
SAM	1.1 ± 0.5	0.5–2.3	0.9 ± 0.5	0.5–2.0	0.242	−0.7–0.2	0.4	Small

BMI: Body Mass Index; SD: standard deviation; min: minimum; max: maximum; CI: confidence interval; *: statistically significance between male and female rowers ($p < 0.05$).

Figure 2 shows the associations between anthropometric variables and rowing performance expressed in mean power output reached in 2000 m rowing test. The results show a strong correlation with body mass in male rowers ($r = 0.57$; $p = 0.021$) and a very strong correlation in female rowers ($r = 0.70$; $p = 0.009$). However, height was strongly correlated in female rowers ($r = 0.64$; $p = 0.017$) and very strongly correlated in male rowers ($r = 0.75$; $p = 0.002$) with performance. Finally, a very strong correlation was found between rowing performance and muscle mass in female rowers ($r = 0.83$; $p = 0.001$), while in male rowers the correlation was small ($r = 0.42$; $p = 0.075$).

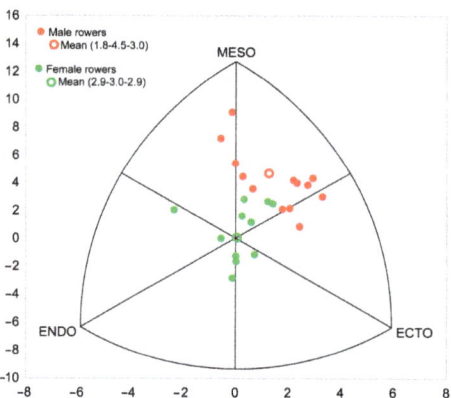

Figure 1. Somatochart of male and female rowers and mean somatotypes.

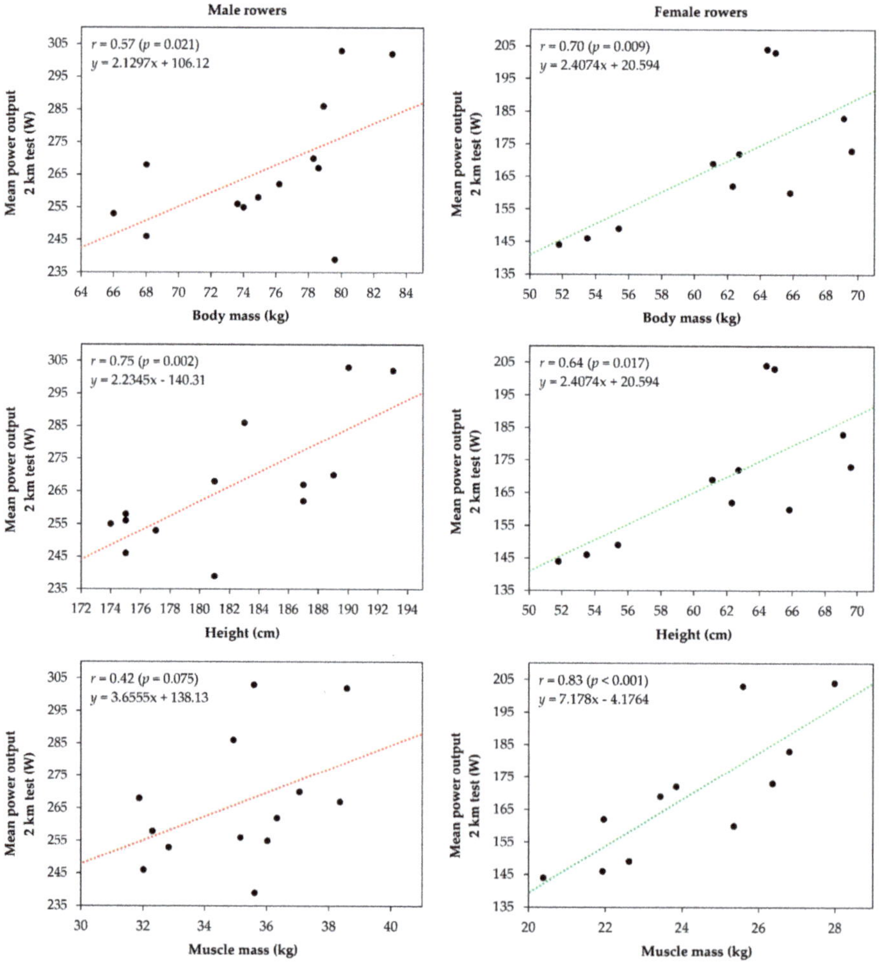

Figure 2. Relationships between anthropometric characteristics and rowing performance in male and female rowers.

Table 3 shows the results of the stepwise multiple regression analysis in male and female rowers by which height is the only predictor of rowing performance in male rowers, explaining 56% of variance ($R^2 = 0.56$, $p < 0.003$). The single predictor of rowing performance in female rowers was muscle mass, explaining explained 68% of variance ($R^2 = 0.68$, $p < 0.002$). The rest of anthropometric measures did not contribute significatively and were excluded from the prediction equation.

Table 3. Stepwise multiple regression model of rowing performance.

Rowers	Equation	R^2	Adj. R^2	SEE	p
Male	$W_{2000m} = 2.23 \times$ Height (cm) $- 140.31$	0.56	0.52	13.72	0.003
Female	$W_{2000m} = 7.18 \times$ Muscle mass (kg) $- 4.18$	0.68	0.65	12.28	0.002

SEE: standard error of estimate; W: power.

4. Discussion

The aim of this study was to analyze and compare the anthropometric profile, body composition, and somatotype in male and female traditional rowers. In addition, the present study aimed to analyze which variables can be used as predictors of rowing performance. As it is the first study that compares the anthropometric profile of traditional rowing between male and female rowers to determine reliable reference values, the selection criteria of the participants were to have classified for the national championship, to have an experience of at least 3 years and to regularly train a minimum of six days per week for 2–3 h/day.

The anthropometric measurements of our study showed that body mass and height mean values were higher in male rowers (182.1 ± 6.6 cm, 75.3 ± 5.3 kg) than female rowers (169.9 ± 6.7 cm, body mass: 61.9 ± 6.0 kg). Results also showed that height and body mass correlate with rowing performance in male and female rowers. Furthermore, height was the best predictor of performance in male rowers ($R^2 = 0.56$, $p < 0.003$). Although there is no scientific evidence on studies of comparative analysis of a complete body composition profile between male and female rowers in traditional rowing, some of the rowers' characteristics in studies on traditional rowing are consistent with this study. Elite traditional male rowers from the Spanish First League of Traineras (ACT) showed a very similar body mass and height to our male rowers (77.0 ± 7.6 kg and 181.1 ± 3.4 cm) [37]. However, other studies have indicated that elite traditional male rowers were heavier (84.4 ± 6.3 kg) but with similar height (182.5 ± 5.2 kg) [8]. In other studies, traditional male rowers of lower competitive level were shorter (178.4 ± 8.9 cm) but with similar body mass (77.3 ± 7.9 kg) [26]. The winners of the Traineras women's league and the La Concha championship [38] coincide with height (168.2 ± 6.3 cm) and body mass (61.2 ± 4.4 kg) results of our study. However, female rowers in Sebastiá-Amat et al. [26] were slightly shorter (166.3 ± 7.5 kg) and lighter (59.9 ± 8.3 cm). It is generally accepted that height is a very important anthropometric characteristic for rowing performance because a greater height increases the amplitude of the drive in the water [7,39]. The results of the studies on Olympic rowing follow the same trend in both height and body mass. Male Olympic rowers reach heights over 190 cm and weigh more than 90 kg, while female rowers exceed 180 cm in height with a body mass of around 75 kg [14,18,19,40]. These discrepancies may be because the height of rowers can be a differentiating characteristic between higher and lower performance in traditional modalities, while the same does not happen with body mass. However, the rowers of the Trainera boat seem to have a higher average weight than the Llaüt rowers. This may be due to the difference in the number of rowers in each boat and the need for the bow rowers to be lighter, lowering the average weight in the Llaüt for correct navigation. Several studies suggest that traditional rowing boats require rowers with different anthropometric profiles, especially in the bow, due to the hydrodynamics of the boat when competitions are held at sea and the body mass placement of the rowers is important [2,8,38].

In the same way, BMI has reached higher values in male rowers (22.8 ± 1.3 kg/m^2) than in female rowers (21.4 ± 1.0 kg/m^2). Studies about male traditional rowers have shown values of BMI greater than 23 kg/m^2 [34,37] and 24 kg/m^2 [7,8,26]. However, BMI of our male rowers is similar to lightweight Olympic (22.1 ± 0.3 kg/m^2) since the rowers in the present study weighed less than the rowers in both traditional and Olympic rowing studies. Finally, BMI values of our female rowers were similar to other traditional rowing (21.7 ± 2.6 kg/m^2) [26] and Olympic rowing studies (21.6 ± 6.1 kg/m^2) [19]. In this latest study, Winkert et al. suggested a body composition with high lean body mass and adequate power to body mass ratios instead of a high body mass, because increased body mass and BMI showed a negative effect on career attainment.

The skinfolds and mean of the sum of 8 skinfolds have a larger value in female rowers (88.0 ± 17.6 mm) than in male rowers (58.5 ± 12.4 mm). It is important to know the values obtained from the skinfold measurement, as it is used to predict fat mass. Furthermore, these differences were expected because women have 6 to 11 percent more body fat than men. Studies show that estrogens reduce a woman's ability to burn energy after eating, thus storing more fat in the body [41]. However, female rowers have lower values in girths and breadths, both in the upper body and in the lower body, except for hip girths with very little difference. In contrast to the scientific literature, it seems that the male rowers in our study have lower values in the sum of skinfolds (67.3 ± 15.6 mm) compared to elite traditional rowers [8]. Compared to rowers participating in the 2000 Sydney Olympic Games [18], the sum of skinfolds of the male rowers in the present study is between open-class (65.3 ± 17.3 mm) and lightweight (44.7 ± 8.1 mm). In the case of female traditional rowers, the values are very similar to the values reached by the open-class female rowers (89.0 ± 23.6 mm). The sum of skinfolds of the lightweight female rowers was only 59.7 ± 12.4 mm.

In our study, male traditional rowers have similar values of muscle mass (46.7 ± 2.0%) compared to other traditional rowing studies of competitions of the same distance as the present study: 46.5 ± 2.0% [34], and large values than other studies of competitions over much longer distances where slimmer rowers are needed.: 43.5 ± 2.0% [42] 43.3 ± 2.4% [8]. According to other studies, female rowers achieved a lower percentage of muscle mass (39.1 ± 2.1%). However, muscle mass for female rowers may be a good predictor of performance in traditional rowing in our study (R^2 = 0.68, $p < 0.002$) and in the scientific literature [26]. This may be because women have much less testosterone than men and due to the influence of this hormone on the development of strength and muscles, women are less likely to develop equal strength and muscle size than men [43]. Therefore, the difference in strength between women is greater than between men and this characteristic seems to become a differentiating factor in performance. In female rowers. On the other hand, female rowers achieved higher fat mass (15.4 ± 3.1%) than male rowers (10.3 ± 2.1%), according to the description of elite rowers of González [38], where female rowers reached 16.3 ± 5.5% and male rowers 7.8 ± 1.1%. Studies on elite male rowers showed lower percentages of fat mass (9.9 ± 2.0%) [8] than studies conducted with sub-elite rowers (14.2 ± 4.4%) [25]. The percentage ranges for international Olympic rowers was 6% to 10% and 11% to 15% for male and female, respectively [44].

In the only two studies published to date on anthropometric profile of traditional male rowers, endo-mesomorph somatotypes were found (3.5-4.7-2.4 [8] and 3.3-3.9-2.2 [42]). However, the mean somatotype in the present study is categorized as ecto-mesomorph (1.8-4.5-3.0) for male rowers, and balanced mesomorph (2.9-3.1-2.9) for female rowers following Carter and Heath [33] where in ecto-mesomorph somatotype, the mesomorphy component is dominant and the ectomorphy component is greater than the endomorphy component; and in balanced mesomorph somatotype, the mesomorphy component is dominant and the endomorphy and ectomorphy components are equal. Our results coincide with the results of Olympic rowers where male rowers had a somatotype defined as ecto-mesomorph (1.9-5.0-2.5) and female rowers a somatotype categorized as balanced mesomorph (2.8-3.8-2.6). The difference between studies may be due to the competition distances of the rowers analyzed from each study: 14,816 m [42] and 5556 m [8]. On the other hand, the rowers in the present study had to row over 1400 m, a distance much more like the 2000 m that Olympic rowers must cover.

Results of the present study should be interpreted with caution because the main limitation of this study lies in the sample size. Also, some of the results are the product of predictive equations rather than direct measurements. Therefore, they can be used as references but should be interpreted in the context of individual characteristics and needs. In addition, it is important to bear in mind that the evaluations have been individual and on rowing ergometer, while the athletes compete in collective boats that may require different profiles as mentioned above. Future research should analyze the differences by position in the boat: bow, stern, and rest rowers. The need for more heterogeneous rowers in traditional rowing boats compared to Olympic rowing may yield a more detailed profile by position. Furthermore, it would be interesting to determine the relationships between the anthropometric profile and rowing performance in male and female traditional rowers to define which characteristics might be most relevant to each one.

5. Conclusions

This study analyzed and compared the anthropometric profile, body composition, and somatotype in male and female traditional rowers, and the role of these variables in the prediction of rowing performance. The results showed that male traditional rowers were significantly taller and heavier, with higher values of girths and breadths, in addition to greater muscle mass. Female traditional rowers reached higher sum of skinfolds and greater fat mass. The mean somatotype for male and female traditional rowers was ecto-mesomorph and balanced mesomorph, respectively, with significant differences in the mesomorph region of male rowers and the endomorph region of female rowers.

Large values of body mass and height correlated with rowing performance in male and female rowers, highlighting height as the best predictor of rowing performance for male traditional rowers. Furthermore, muscle mass positively correlated in female rowers, being the best predictor for rowing performance.

This study shows a detailed anthropometric description of traditional rowers competing at the national level that can be useful as reference values for coaches and rowers. Furthermore, the study shows different variables that can be used to control training and increase rowing performance, such as body and muscle mass, and to identify potential talents in young athletes thanks to characteristics such as height.

Author Contributions: Conceptualization, A.P.-T., B.P. and J.M.J.-O.; Formal analysis, S.S.-P.; Investigation, A.P.-T., B.P. and J.M.J.-O.; Methodology, A.P.-T., B.P., S.S.-P. and J.M.J.-O.; Resources, S.S.-P. and J.M.J.-O.; Supervision, B.P.; Writing—original draft, A.P.-T.; Writing—review & editing, A.P.-T., B.P., S.S.-P. and J.M.J.-O. All authors have read and agreed to the published version of the manuscript.

Funding: This research received no external funding.

Institutional Review Board Statement: The study was conducted according to the guidelines of the Declaration of Helsinki and approved by the Institutional Review Board of University of Alicante (IRB No. UA-2020-07-21, date of approval: 8 August 2020).

Informed Consent Statement: Written informed consent was obtained from all subjects involved in the study.

Data Availability Statement: The data presented in this study are available on reasonable request from the corresponding author.

Conflicts of Interest: The authors declare no conflict of interest.

References

1. Lorenzo Buceta, H.; Pérez Treus, S.; García Soidán, J.L.; Arufe Giraldez, V.; Cornes, X.A.; Cornes, A.A. Dynamic analysis on the fixed seat rowing: Trainera. *Retos* **2014**, *2041*, 120–123.
2. Baudouin, A.; Hawkins, D. A biomechanical review of factors affecting rowing performance. *Br. J. Sports Med.* **2002**, *36*, 396–402. [CrossRef]

3. Lorenzo-Buceta, H.; García-Soidán, J.L. Dynamic response analysis of a rowing fixed boat bank (trainerilla) by the application of accelerometry. *J. Sport Health Res.* **2015**, *7*, 55–64.
4. Kleshnev, V. *Biomechanics of Rowing*; The Crowood Press: Ramsbury, UK, 2016.
5. Cerasola, D.; Bellafiore, M.; Cataldo, A.; Zangla, D.; Bianco, A.; Proia, P.; Traina, M.; Palma, A.; Capranica, L. Predicting the 2000-m rowing ergometer performance from anthropometric, maximal oxygen uptake and 60-s mean power variables in national level young rowers. *J. Hum. Kinet.* **2020**, *75*, 77–83. [CrossRef]
6. Penichet-tomas, A.; Pueo, B.; Abad-lopez, M.; Jimenez-olmedo, J.M. Acute comparative effect of foam rolling and static stretching on range of motion in rowers. *Sustainability* **2021**, *13*, 3631. [CrossRef]
7. Penichet-Tomás, A.; Pueo, B.; Jiménez-Olmedo, J. Physical performance indicators in traditional rowing championships. *J. Sports Med. Phys. Fit.* **2019**, *59*, 767–773. [CrossRef]
8. León-Guereño, P.; Urdampilleta, A.; Zourdos, M.C.; Mielgo-Ayuso, J. Anthropometric profile, body composition and somatotype in elite traditional rowers: A cross-sectional study. *Rev. Española Nutr. Diet.* **2018**, *2*, 279–286. [CrossRef]
9. González, J.M. Olympic rowing and traditional rowing: Biomechanical, physiological and nutritional aspects. *Arch. Med. Deporte* **2014**, *31*, 51–59.
10. De Larochelambert, Q.; Del Vecchio, S.; Leroy, A.; Duncombe, S.; Toussaint, J.-F.; Sedeaud, A. Body and Boat: Significance of Morphology on Elite Rowing Performance. *Front. Sports Act. Living* **2020**, *2*. [CrossRef] [PubMed]
11. Akça, F. Prediction of rowing ergometer performance from functional anaerobic power, strength and anthropometric components. *J. Hum. Kinet.* **2014**, *41*, 133–142. [CrossRef]
12. Izquierdo-Gabarren, M.; González, R.; Sáez, E.; Izquierdo, M. Physiological factors to predict on traditional rowing performance. *Eur. J. Appl. Physiol.* **2010**, *108*, 83–92. [CrossRef]
13. Kaloupsis, S.; Bogdanis, G.C.; Dimakopoulou, E.; Maridaki, M. Anthropometric characteristics and somatotype of young Greek rowers. *Biol. Sport* **2008**, *25*, 57–69.
14. Mikulić, P. Anthropometric and physiological profiles of rowers of varying ages and ranks. *Kinesiology* **2008**, *40*, 80–88.
15. Gutiérrez-Leyton, L.; Zavala-Crichton, J.; Fuentes-Toledo, C.; Yáñez-Sepúlveda, R. Anthropometric characteristics and somatotype in elite Chilean rowers. *Int. J. Morphol.* **2020**, *38*, 114–119. [CrossRef]
16. Arslanoğlu, E.; Acar, K.; Mor, A.; Baynaz, K.; İpekoğlu, G.; Arslanoglu, C. Body composition and somatotype profiles of rowers. *Turk. J. Sport Exerc.* **2020**, *22*, 431–437. [CrossRef]
17. Adhikari, A.; McNeely, E. Anthropometric characteristic, somatotype and body composition of Canadian female rowers. *Am. J. Sports Sci.* **2015**, *3*, 61–66. [CrossRef]
18. Kerr, D.A.; Ross, W.D.; Norton, K.; Hume, P.; Kagawa, M.; Ackland, T.R. Olympic lightweight and open-class rowers possess distinctive physical and proportionality characteristics. *J. Sports Sci.* **2007**, *25*, 43–53. [CrossRef] [PubMed]
19. Winkert, K.; Steinacker, J.M.; Machus, K.; Dreyhaupt, J.; Treff, G. Anthropometric profiles are associated with long-term career attainment in elite junior rowers: A retrospective analysis covering 23 years. *Eur. J. Sport Sci.* **2019**, *19*, 208–216. [CrossRef] [PubMed]
20. Schranz, N.; Tomkinson, G.; Olds, T.; Daniell, N. Three-dimensional anthropometric analysis: Differences between elite Australian rowers and the general population. *J. Sports Sci.* **2010**, *28*, 459–469. [CrossRef] [PubMed]
21. Yoshiga, C.C.; Higuchi, M. Rowing performance of female and male rowers. *Scand. J. Med. Sci. Sports* **2003**, *13*, 317–321. [CrossRef]
22. Ingham, S.; Whyte, G.; Jones, K.; Nevill, A. Determinants of 2,000 m rowing ergometer performance in elite rowers. *Eur. J. Appl. Physiol.* **2002**, *88*, 243–246. [CrossRef]
23. Mikulic, P. Anthropometric and metabolic determinants of 6000-m rowing ergometer performance in internationally competitive rowers. *J. Strength Cond. Res.* **2009**, *23*, 1851–1857. [CrossRef]
24. Campa, F.; Toselli, S.; Mazzilli, M.; Gobbo, L.A.; Coratella, G. Assessment of body composition in athletes: A narrative review of available methods with special reference to quantitative and qualitative bioimpedance analysis. *Nutrients* **2021**, *13*, 1620. [CrossRef] [PubMed]
25. Mejuto, G.; Arratibel, I.; Cámara, J.; Puente, A.; Iturriaga, G.; Calleja-González, J. The effect of a 6-week individual anaerobic threshold based programme in a traditional rowing crew. *Biol. Sport* **2012**, *29*, 297–301. [CrossRef]
26. Sebastia-Amat, S.; Penichet-Tomas, A.; Jimenez-Olmedo, J.M.; Pueo, B. Contributions of anthropometric and strength determinants to estimate 2000 m ergometer performance in traditional rowing. *Appl. Sci.* **2020**, *10*, 6562. [CrossRef]
27. Ross, W.D.; Marfell-Jones, M.J. Kinanthropometry. In *Physiological Testing of Elite Athlete*; Human Kinetics Publishers Inc.: London, UK, 1991; pp. 223–308.
28. Pueo, B.; Espina-Agullo, J.J.; Selles-Perez, S.; Penichet-Tomas, A. Optimal body composition and anthropometric profile of world-class beach handball players by playing positions. *Sustainability* **2020**, *12*, 6789. [CrossRef]
29. Sellés-Pérez, S.; García-Jaén, M.; Cortell-Tormo, J.M.; Cejuela, R. A short-term body jump® training program improves physical fitness and body composition in young active women. *Appl. Sci.* **2021**, *11*, 3234. [CrossRef]
30. Withers, R.T.; Craig, N.P.; Bourdon, P.C.; Norton, K.I. Relative body fat and anthropometric prediction of body density of male athletes. *Eur. J. Appl. Physiol. Occup. Physiol.* **1987**, *56*, 191–200. [CrossRef] [PubMed]
31. Lee, R.C.; Wang, Z.; Heo, M.; Ross, R.; Janssen, I.; Heymsfield, S.B. Total-body skeletal muscle mass: Development and cross-validation of anthropometric prediction models. *Am. J. Clin. Nutr.* **2000**, *72*, 796–803. [CrossRef]
32. Rocha, M. Peso ósseo do brasileiro de ambos os sexos de 17 a 25 anos. *Arq. Anatomía Antropol.* **1975**, *1*, 445–451.

33. Carter, J.E.; Heath, B.H. *Somatotyping—Development and Applications*; Cambridge University Press: New York, NY, USA, 1990.
34. Penichet-Tomas, A.; Jimenez-Olmedo, J.M.; Serra Torregrosa, L.; Pueo, B. Acute effects of different postactivation potentiation protocols on traditional rowing performance. *Int. J. Environ. Res. Public Health* **2021**, *18*, 80. [CrossRef] [PubMed]
35. Cohen, J. *Statistical Power Analysis for the Behavioral Sciences*; Lawrence E.: Mahwah, NJ, USA, 1988; ISBN 0805802835.
36. Hopkins, W.G. A Scale of Magnitudes for the Effect Statistics. A New View of Statistics. Available online: http://www.sportsci.org/resource/stats/ (accessed on 13 February 2021).
37. Mielgo-Ayuso, J.; Calleja-González, J.; Urdampilleta, A.; León-Guereño, P.; Córdova, A.; Caballero-García, A.; Fernandez-Lázaro, D. Effects of vitamin D supplementation on haematological values and muscle recovery in elite male traditional rowers. *Nutrients* **2018**, *10*, 1968. [CrossRef] [PubMed]
38. González, J.M. Remo olímpico y remo tradicional: Aspectos biomecánicos, fisiológicos y nutricionales. *Arch. Med. Deporte* **2014**, *159*, 51–59.
39. Mujika, I.; González, R.; Maldonado-Martín, S.; Pyne, D.B. Warm-up intensity and duration's effect on traditional rowing time-trial performance. *Int. J. Sports Physiol. Perform.* **2012**, *7*, 186–188. [CrossRef]
40. Rakovac, M.; Smoljanovic, T.; Bojanic, I.; Hannafin, J.A.; Hren, D.; Thomas, P. Body size changes in elite junior rowers: 1997 to 2007. *Coll. Antropol.* **2011**, *35*, 127–131.
41. O'Sullivan, A.J. Does oestrogen allow women to store fat more efficiently? A biological advantage for fertility and gestation. *Obes. Rev.* **2009**, *10*, 168–177. [CrossRef]
42. Cejuela, R.; Pérez-Turpin, J.A.; Cortell, J.M.; Llopis, J.; Chinchilla, J.J. An analysis of performance in long-distance rowing by means of global positioning system technology. *Int. J. Comput. Sci. Sport* **2008**, *7*, 59–65.
43. Wood, R.I.; Stanton, S.J. Testosterone and sport: Current perspectives. *Horm. Behav.* **2012**, *61*, 147–155. [CrossRef]
44. Arazi, H.; Faraji, H.; Mohammadi, S.M. Anthropometric and physiological profiles of elite Iranian junior rowers. *Middle-East J. Sci. Res.* **2011**, *9*, 162–166.

Article

Bioimpedance Vector Patterns according to Age and Handgrip Strength in Adolescent Male and Female Athletes

Marcus Vinicius de Oliveira Cattem [1], Bruna Taranto Sinforoso [1], Francesco Campa [2] and Josely Correa Koury [1,*]

1. Department of Basic and Experimental Nutrition, Nutrition Institute, State University of Rio de Janeiro, Rio de Janeiro 20550-900, Brazil; mv_cattem@hotmail.com (M.V.d.O.C.); bruna.taranto@nutricao.ufrj.br (B.T.S.)
2. Department for Life Quality Studies, University of Bologna, 47921 Rimini, Italy; francesco.campa3@unibo.it
* Correspondence: jckoury@gmail.com

Abstract: Bioelectric Impedance Vector Analysis (BIVA) can be used to qualitatively compare individuals' hydration and cell mass independently of predictive equations. This study aimed to analyze the efficiency of BIVA considering chronological age and handgrip strength in adolescent athletes. A total of 273 adolescents (male; 59%) engaged in different sports were evaluated. Bioelectrical impedance (Z), resistance (R), reactance (Xc), and phase angle (PhA) were obtained using a single-frequency bioelectrical impedance analyzer. Fat-free mass (FFM) and total body water were estimated using bioimpedance-based equations specific for adolescents. Female showed higher values of R (5.5%, $p = 0.001$), R/height (3.8%, $p = 0.041$), Z (5.3%, $p = 0.001$), and fat mass (53.9%, $p = 0.001$) than male adolescents. Male adolescents showed higher values of FFM (5.3%, $p = 0.021$) and PhA (3.1%, $p = 0.033$) than female adolescents. In both stratifications, adolescents (older > 13 years or stronger > median value) shifted to the left on the R-Xc graph, showing patterns of higher hydration and cell mass. The discrimination of subjects older than 13 years and having higher median of handgrip strength values was possibly due to maturity differences. This study showed that BIVA identified age and strength influence in vector displacement, assessing qualitative information and offering patterns of vector distribution in adolescent athletes.

Keywords: adolescent athletes; body composition; BIVA; confidence ellipses; fat-free mass; R-Xc graph; tolerance ellipses

1. Introduction

Strenuous training could be a matter for the competitive adolescent athletes, since high intensity and high training volume impose nutritional and functional risks to body development [1]. Exercise practice has been associated with the development of bone [2] and muscle tissues [3]. Fat-free mass (FFM) is considered a predictor of muscle strength and physical capacities [4–7]. Assessments of body composition contribute to verify the effects of physical activity and sports practice over time.

Muscle strength is another valuable measurement in physically active individuals as it impacts sports performance, daily activities, life quality and is related to low incidence and prevalence of diseases [8]. In order to assess handgrip strength, handgrip dynamometers are easy to use, simple, and not expensive [9]. Muscle strength is also related to gender, chronological and biological age, and body composition, since FFM is important to produce it and fat mass (FM) may limit it in contact sports, for example [10,11]. Handgrip strength has been used in youth soccer and female basketball players for talent identification [12,13].

Bioelectrical Impedance Analysis (BIA) can be used as a non-invasive method to estimate FFM, FM, and total body water (TBW) from electrical body proprieties of resistance (R) and reactance (Xc) while considering individual characteristics, such as sex, age, height, and weight [14,15]. BIA presents good correlation and concordance with dual energy X-ray absorptiometry (DXA) also when analyzing adolescent athletes [16]. However, BIA equations are dependent on specific characteristics of the population [15]. For this reason, in recent years, Bioelectric Impedance Vector Analysis (BIVA) has gained relevance for sports [17,18], because its qualitative and semi-quantitative analysis of impedance vectors and impedance components are directly plotted on the R-Xc graph. BIVA graphics are interpreted by impedance vector lengths and their ellipses and phase angle (PhA) [19]. PhA is derived from R and Xc, and it has been interpreted as an index of membrane integrity and water distribution between intra and extracellular compartments [20]. In addition, PhA has been used as a predictor of body cell mass, and for this reason, it has been employed as an indicator of nutritional status [21]. The complementary use of the BIVA and PhA may be helpful in the evaluation of changes of nutrition and hydration status in athletes [22].

Moreover, BIVA provides qualitative information of soft tissue classification and ranking, comparing individual vectors and ellipses to reference populations [23]. In this context, it is important to develop BIVA references for adolescent athletes considering handgrip strength. To the best of our knowledge, there are no studies that relate BIVA and handgrip strength in female and male adolescent athletes.

Considering the importance of body composition and strength to sports practice and for adolescent health, and considering BIVA a useful tool to assess adolescent athletes, the aim of this study was to analyze the efficiency of BIVA, considering chronological age and handgrip strength in female and male adolescent athletes.

2. Materials and Methods

2.1. Study Design and Subjects

This was a cross-sectional observational study. Two hundred and seventy-three Brazilian healthy adolescents (n = 161, males [59%]), aged mean 12.9 ± 0.9 years participated. All the data were collected at a sports-oriented public school located in the central region of the city of Rio de Janeiro, Brazil (2012–2013). This is an elementary full-time school that, unlike other public schools, offers 120 min of daily sports training and seven sports modalities: swimming, judo, badminton, athletics, soccer, volleyball, and table tennis, in which the students practiced different sports for the same amount of time.

The adolescents were classified as athletes, because they participated in training, skill development, and were engaged in competition, according to the definition described in Sports Dietitians Australia Position Statement: Sports nutrition for the adolescent athletes [24].

The participants were classified according to sex, handgrip strength (high—above median value; low—under median value) and chronological age ($\leq$13 or >13 years). In adolescents, body composition is highly interrelated to biological maturity, due to hormones and growth factors function [1]. In the absence of consistent maturation indicators, adolescents can be divided into $\leq$13 and >13 years [25]. Mathias-Genovez et al. (2016) [26] showed that in the Brazilian adolescent population, 13 years was the age at which changes in body composition start due to biological maturation.

An a priori power analysis was conducted to determine the sample size using statistical software (G*Power v. 3.1.9.2, Stuttgart, Germany). The sample size calculation was performed assuming the values of r = 40%, α = 5%, and β = 20%, so the number of students estimated by each sex was 126. However, at the end of the study, 161 male and 112 female adolescents participated.

To participate in this study, adolescents and parents agreed to participate after a full explanation of the research objectives. This study was approved by the Ethics Committee of the Pedro Ernesto Hospital (CEP/HUPE 1.020.909).

2.2. Anthropometric and Body Composition Measurements

Weight was measured with a portable scale to the nearest 0.1 kg (Filizola, Brazil), height was measured with a stadiometer to the nearest 0.5 cm (Sanny, Brazil), and Body Mass Index (BMI = weight[kg]/height^2[m]) was calculated.

BIA measurements were always performed in the morning, using a tetrapolar analyzer RJL (Quantum 101; Systems, Clinton Township, MI USA), which applies an alternating current of 800 µA at a single frequency of 50 kHz. Participants were in the supine position with a leg opening distant 45° from the median line of the body and the upper limbs distant 30° from the trunk. Electrodes were applied on the right wrist and ankle after cleansing the skin with alcohol in a thermo-neutral environment of 25 °C. To avoid disturbances in fluid distribution, participants were instructed to abstain from foods and liquids for at least 4 h as well as refrain from caffeine intake and intense physical activity 24 h prior to the BIA analysis. Before each testing session, the analyzer was checked with a calibration circuit of known impedance (resistance = 500.0 Ω; reactance = 0.1 Ω; 0.9% error). Resistance (R) and reactance (Xc) were used to calculate phase angle (PhA) [20]. FFM and total body water were assessed using a predictive equation developed by Horlick et al. [27]. The BIA predictive equations used in this study are listed in Table 1. Fat mass (FM) was calculated subtracting FFM from weight, and fat mass percentage was calculated by (FM/weight) × 100.

Table 1. Predictive equations used in the present study.

	Equations	Reference
Phase angle	=arc tangent (Xc/R) × (180°/π)	Baumgartner et al. [20]
Fat-free mass	=[3.474 + 0.459*H²/R + 0.064 × Wt]/[0.769 − 0.009*age − 0.016 × sex]	Horlick et al. [27]
Total body water	=0.725 + 0.475 × H²/R + 0.140 × Wt	Horlick et al. [27]

H = height (cm); Wt = weight (kg); R = resistance; Xc = reactance; sex = 0 for females and 1 for males.

2.3. Handgrip Strength

Handgrip strength was assessed with a hand JAMAR-dynamometer (Asimow Engineering Co., Los Angeles, CA, USA) in both hands alternately, three times, and the mean value was recorded to obtain a single value of HG.

2.4. Bioelectrical Impedance Vector Analysis

BIVA was developed based on the R and Xc vectors normalized by height (H) [19,28]. The experimental data are plotted in the R-Xc graph and compared with the 95th-percentile confidence ellipses from a reference population. The correlation between R and Xc determines the ellipsoidal form of the bivariate probability distributions [28].

BIVA tolerance consists of plotting the experimental data in a bivariate graph considering the 95th, 75th, and 50th vector percentiles of the Z-score of the reference population. Considering the plotting position of the experimental data, it is possible to suggest an interpretation: abnormal situation, when experimental data are positioned outside of the 95th percentile ellipsis; higher body cell mass, when experimental data are located above the long axis of the ellipsis; hypohydration, when experimental data are positioned to the right of the short axis of the ellipsis. Total body water is inversely related to the length of the impedance vector, and a combination of the vector length and its direction is defined as PhA [28,29] (Figure 1). The reference population for adolescents used in the BIVA analyses was obtained from the dataset of Koury et al. [16].

2.5. Statistical Analysis

All analyses were performed separately for each sex, and participants were classified according to chronological age ($\leq$ 3 or >13 years) and handgrip strength median. Continuous variables were expressed as mean and standard deviation. An independent t-test followed by the Bonferroni post hoc test was used to compare variables between chronological ages. A linear regression model assessed the relation between handgrip strength (outcome) and chronological age, fat-free mass, and PhA (predictors). Univariate linear regression with backward stepwise elimination results were presented as unstandardized B coefficients, 95% confidence intervals (CI), and p-value. p-value < 0.05 was considered statistically significant. All statistical analyses were performed using STATISTICA 10 software (Stat Soft. Inc., Tulsa, OK, USA).

For BIVA, the two-sample Hotelling T^2 test was used to compare differences in mean impedance vectors in BIVA confidence analyses, and the Mahalanobis test was used to calculate the distances between ellipses. Confidence and the 50%, 75%, and 95% tolerance ellipses were generated using BIVA software [29].

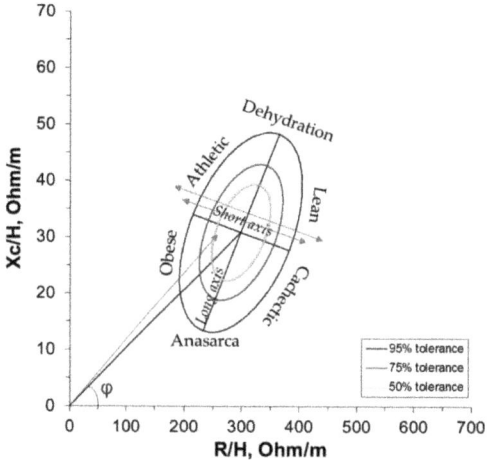

Figure 1. BIVA nomogram pattern, RXc-graph. Resistance (R) and reactance (Xc) were normalized by the height (H, meter) (adapted from Piccoli and Pastore, 2002).

3. Results

Characteristics of the adolescent athletes according to sex and chronological age are shown in Table 2. Female adolescents showed higher values of R (5.5%, $p < 0.01$), R/H (3.8%, $p = 0.041$), Z (5.3%, $p < 0.01$), and fat mass (53.9%, $p < 0.01$) than male adolescents. Male adolescents showed higher values of FFM (5.3%, $p = 0.021$) and PhA (3.1%, $p = 0.033$) than female adolescents. According to chronological age, older female adolescents showed higher values of weight (19.9%, $p < 0.01$), height (3.2%, $p < 0.01$), BMI (13.5%, $p < 0.01$), PhA (5.1%, $p = 0.002$), FFM (14.9%, $p < 0.01$), FM (37.5%, $p < 0.01$), TBW (15%, $p < 0.01$), and handgrip strength (17.5%, $p < 0.01$). In addition to that, older female adolescents showed lower values of R (6.9%, $p < 0.01$), R/H (10.5%, $p < 0.01$), and Z (6.8%, $p = 0.002$) than younger participants. Older male adolescents showed higher values of weight (17.2%, $p < 0.01$), height (7.3%, $p < 0.01$), FFM (22.2%, $p < 0.01$), TBW (21.5%, $p < 0.01$), and handgrip strength (35.2%, $p < 0.01$); they showed lower values of R (7.5%, $p < 0.01$), R/H (15.3%, $p < 0.01$), Xc (8.9%, $p < 0.01$), Xc/H (16.4%, $p < 0.01$), and Z (7.7%, $p < 0.01$) than younger male adolescents. The different modalities practiced did not present any significant difference in the results of body composition and age.

Handgrip strength values are shown according to sex and chronological age (≤ 13.0 or >13.0 years) in Figure 2. The median value of handgrip strength was used to stratify female and male participants in groups of low and high handgrip strength. Individuals up to the median of handgrip strength of their sex were classified as low handgrip strength and individuals above the median were classified as high handgrip strength. The median of the female group was 20.6 kgf and that of the male group was 21.1 kgf. Differences were found between older and younger individuals of the same sex ($p = 0.01$) and between male and female participants at older age ($p = 0.02$), but not between younger subjects.

Table 2. Descriptive and comparative general characteristics, according to sex and age categories ($n = 273$).

Characteristics	All			Age (Years)						
				Female			Male			
	Female	Male	p	≤13.0	>13.0	p	≤13.0	>13.0	p	
n	112	161		59	53		101	60		
Age (years)	13.0 ± 0.9	12.8 ± 0.9	0.183	12.25 ± 0.46	13.82 ± 0.55	<0.01	12.28 ± 0.42	13.81 ± 0.50	<0.01	
Weight (kg)	51.1 ± 10.1	48.9 ± 11.5	0.098	46.7 ± 9.9	56.0 ± 8.0	<0.01	45.9 ± 10.8	53.8 ± 10.9	<0.01	
Height (cm)	157.7 ± 7.4	156.1 ± 9.9	0.153	155.3 ± 6.8	160.3 ± 7.2	<0.01	152.0 ± 7.9 **	163.1 ± 9.0	<0.01	
BMI (kg/m^2)	20.5 ± 3.4	19.8 ± 3.2	0.124	19.2 ± 3.1	21.8 ± 3.2	<0.01	19.7 ± 3.4	20.1 ± 2.8 **	0.446	
R (Ω)	624.1 ± 70.2	591.7 ± 72.5	<0.01	643.8 ± 70.3	602.2 ± 63.8	<0.01	607.6 ± 72.6 **	565 ± 64.5 **	<0.01	
R/H (Ω/m)	396.9 ± 50.4	382.2 ± 62.9	0.041	415.6 ± 51.8	376 ± 39.9	<0.01	402.0 ± 59.4	348.8 ± 54 **	<0.01	
Xc (Ω)	65.7 ± 7.7	64.4 ± 9.2	0.230	65.8 ± 7.6	65.5 ± 7.8	0.836	66.4 ± 9.1	61.0 ± 8.5 **	<0.01	
Xc/H (Ω/m)	41.8 ± 5.4	41.6 ± 7.6	0.851	42.5 ± 5.6	40.9 ± 5.0	0.125	43.9 ± 7.2	37.7 ± 6.6 **	<0.01	
Z (Ω)	627.6 ± 70.2	595.8 ± 73.0	<0.01	647.2 ± 70.4	605.8 ± 63.9	0.002	612.2 ± 73.2 **	568.3 ± 64.5 **	<0.01	
PhA (degree)	6.0 ± 0.7	6.2 ± 0.7	0.033	5.87 ± 0.6	6.24 ± 0.67	0.67	6.24 ± 0.67 ***	6.20 ± 0.83	0.746	
FFM (kg)	38.9 ± 5.4	40.9 ± 8.2	0.021	36.3 ± 4.8	41.7 ± 4.5	<0.01	37.8 ± 6.6	46.2 ± 7.9 ***	<0.01	
FM (kg)	12.2 ± 6.3	7.9 ± 6	<0.01	10.4 ± 5.9	14.3 ± 6.2	<0.01	8.1 ± 6.2 *	7.7 ± 5.8 ***	0.665	
FM (%)	22.7 ± 8.3	15.2 ± 8.7	0.001	20.8 ± 8.1	24.8 ± 8.0	0.010	16.2 ± 9.0 ***	13.4 ± 7.9 ***	0.046	
TBW (L)	27.1 ± 4.1	27.7 ± 5.9	0.371	25.3 ± 3.9	29.1 ± 3.3	<0.01	25.6 ± 5.0	31.1 ± 5.8 *	<0.01	
HG (kgf)	21.0 ± 4.8	22.2 ± 6.5	0.110	19.4 ± 3.9	22.8 ± 5.1	<0.01	19.6 ± 4.9	26.5 ± 6.7 **	<0.01	

BMI: body mass index; R/H: resistance/height ratio; Xc/H: reactance/height ratio; PhA: phase angle; FFM: fat-free mass; FM: fat mass; TBW: total body water; HG: handgrip strength. Intra- and intergroup differences were obtained using an independent t-test followed by the Bonferroni post-hoc test. Significant differences between sexes and the same age category were marked by * ($p < 0.05$), ** ($p < 0.01$), *** ($p < 0.001$).

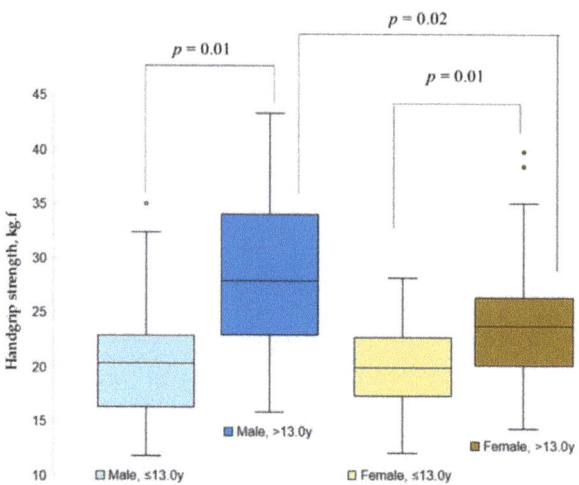

Figure 2. Handgrip strength in female and male according to different age classes (≤13 or >13 years).

Table 3 shows that a linear regression model was applied to verify the influence of chronological age, FFM, PhA, and sex on handgrip strength (outcome). For all participants, chronological age (57.2%; $p = 0.041$) and FFM (62.2%, $p = 0.0001$) could explain the handgrip strength. In the female group, only FFM could explain the model in 56.1% ($p = 0.0001$), and in the male group, chronological age (79.2%, $p = 0.032$) and FFM (63.6%, $p = 0.0001$) could explain the handgrip strength.

Table 3. Handgrip strength independent predictive variables in adolescent athletes.

Variables	All *			Female			Male		
	β	95%CI	p-Value	β	95%CI	p-Value	β	95%CI	p-Value
Chronological age	0.572	0.024–1.119	0.041	0.109	−0.331–1.457	0.215	0.792	0.070–1.513	0.032
Fat-free mass	0.622	0.554–0.690	<0.01	0.561	0.429–0.694	0.001	0.636	0.559–0.714	<0.01
Phase angle	0.058	−0.117–1.087	0.114	0.093	−0.535–1.794	0.245	0.610	−0.093–1.313	0.089

Linear regression model. * adjusted by sex. R^2 all = 0.651, R^2 female = 0.386, R^2 male = 0.753.

Figure 3 shows mean impedance vectors with 95% confidence ellipses for adolescent athletes according to sex and chronological age (Figure 3A) or sex and handgrip strength classification (Figure 3B). Participants showed differences when age and handgrip strength ($p < 0.05$) were compared. Older male and female athletes showed shorter impedance vectors. Similarly, a shorter impedance vector was observed in male and female participants with high handgrip strength. Additionally, when distances between age and handgrip strength ellipses were tested, a significant difference was found only between younger male participants and those with low handgrip strength ($p = 0.033$). In addition, there is a slight overlap in male and female low handgrip strength' ellipses; however, the T^2 test still found a significant difference. Considering age and handgrip strength, 35.6% and 33.7% of the younger female and male adolescents were classified as high handgrip (>median), and 44% and 23.3% of the older individuals were classified as low handgrip strength (<median), respectively.

The data from female (Figure 4A) and male (Figure 4B) adolescent athletes, considering chronological age and handgrip strength classification, were plotted on the BIVA tolerance ellipses of Brazilian adolescent athlete reference population [16]. Both graphs presented a trend of a higher density of points in the 95% tolerance ellipsis. The frequency of points outside the 95% tolerance ellipsis, above the long axis, was 2% for male adolescents and

0.9% for female adolescent athletes. Only one female older and stronger subject was outside the 95% ellipse.

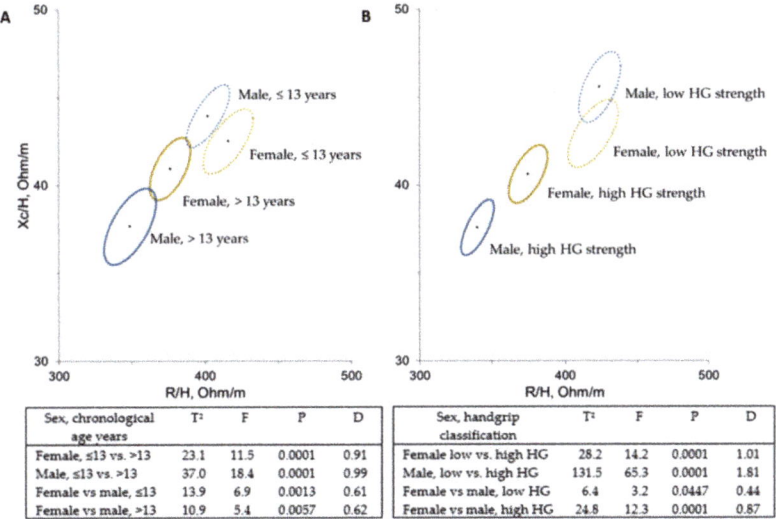

Figure 3. Mean impedance vectors with the 95% confidence ellipses for adolescent athletes sorted by chronological age (**A**) or handgrip strength classification (**B**). Mahalanobis distances (D), Hotelling T^2-tests, F and *p*-values are included.

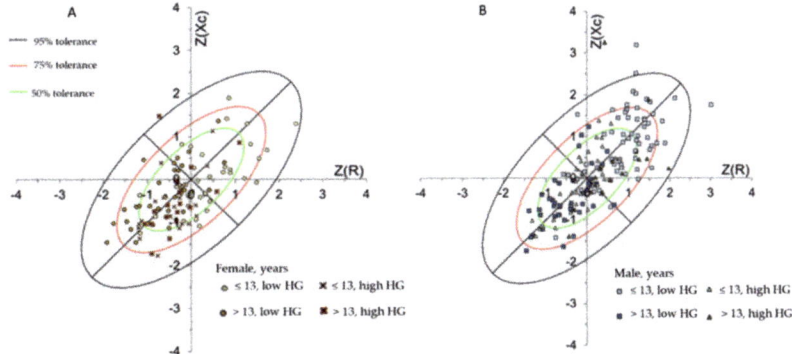

Figure 4. Mean impedance vectors with the 50, 75, and 95% tolerance ellipses for the female (**A**) and male (**B**) adolescent athletes, according to age and handgrip strength categories.

4. Discussion

There is a growing interest in BIVA in sports and physical exercise [17]. The present study shows, for the first time, BIVA patterns from female and male adolescent athletes and their associations with handgrip strength. Only FFM was a predictor of handgrip strength for female and male adolescent athletes. So, higher strength in male adolescents could be explained by the higher FFM throughout male development.

Studies in adolescent athletes are centered in male subjects [30–32]. There is only one study about BIVA in female athletes [23]. The present study is the first that shows BIVA responses associated with strength, brings new references for adolescent athletes, and adds knowledge to this field. Studies such as the present one, which assesses general health, are necessary in order to improve prescription of sports, since it is important to have information on adolescent athletes of both sexes.

Most studies only describe reference values for adult individuals, and thresholds and cutoffs points are needed for all ages and ethnic groups as reviewed by Dodds et al. [33] when analyzing variation in handgrip strength worldwide [33]. In the present study, handgrip strength did not show any statistical difference between female and male adolescents until the age of 13 years. However, it was greater in older male subjects than older female adolescents. In addition, female and male differences accentuated after 13 years of age, which may be attributed to puberty changes [34,35]. FFM/FM proportion may explain the greater strength in older male subjects. FFM is closely related to strength, since FFM is the primary body component that produces it [10]. However, when handgrip strength is standardized by fat-free mass, the difference disappears in this study dataset. Chronological age was important to discriminate male and female individuals by handgrip strength, but it was not a predictor in the linear model in female adolescents.

PhA is often associated with strength and physical fitness in adult athletes [18] and also in male adult and adolescent athletes [31]. PhA was also associated with handgrip strength in healthy adult men [36]. However, this study was conducted in an age range with little PhA variation according to a review of 250,000 subjects in different ages by Mattiello et al. [37]. For this reason, PhA could present a constant behavior in regression models and was not significant in all the analysis. Regarding the role of the somatic maturation on BIVA patterns, Campa et al. [2] identified specific transition periods in which the bioelectrical parameters showed an increase, a decrease, or a plateau. In particular, PhA begins to increase rapidly beginning at two years prior to the maturity offset and continues to do so for the four years following this growth phase [38]. In addition, the vector length shows a sharp decrease up to one year after the maturity offset, which is identifiable with the achievement of the peak height velocity, and then, it reaches a plateau. However, in athletes, the age at peak height velocity can be lower than that measured in the general population [30]. This may represent a common scenario in elite teams, as often there is a tendency to select taller athletes, which is typical in mature adolescents.

BIVA is an effective tool to assess body composition in male and female adult athletes [17,23], although there are no BIVA references to female adolescent athletes and no studies associating BIVA and handgrip strength in adolescent individuals.

In this study with adolescent athletes, BIVA confidence ellipses were sensitive both to age and handgrip strength. Confidence ellipses of older and stronger individuals shifted to the left, indicating increased cell mass and fluid content, which can be attributed to better cell functioning [17], which is consistent with growth development and physical training. It was also noticed that the ellipses of the female group had the same displacement in age and strength categorizations. Ellipses of the male group kept the same general pattern, but there was increased distance in strength categorization.

The hypothesis behind BIVA's greater sensitivity to strength in male adolescents is related to maturity factors, in which the increasing strength is more relevant than chronological age. That means that strength reflects more the increase in body cell mass (especially FFM) and fluid content than age in male individuals. Although there is a slight overlap in both sexes' ellipses in low strength groups, the Hotelling T^2 test was able to identify a significant difference. Since confidence ellipses presented 95% probability, even a slight overlap could not affect the significance of Mahalanobis distance [17]. In this study, from the reference population, tolerance ellipses showed that most individuals were inside the 95% tolerance ellipses. The presence of female adolescents outside the ellipse may be explained by their better training status, which is reflected in higher cell mass; and male adolescents outside the ellipse may be explained by their hypohydration status expressed in long impedance vectors and reinforced by low total body water values ($\leq$50% from weight).

A positive point of this study is a sample size (112 females and 161 males). Additionally, participants were measured in the same physical training conditions. These characteristics are particularly important to BIVA quality and applicability. Some limitations should be acknowledged. First, the present results refer to adolescent athletes and should not be generalized. Second, the bioelectrical parameters were measured using a foot-to-hand technology at 50 kHz frequency and should not be compared with the different technologies or data obtained at different sampling frequencies. Lastly, unfortunately, in the present study, it was not possible to assess the biological maturity status of the participants. However, our results are in agreement with other studies that used chronological age [26,34,39,40] and maturity status [32,38]. Deuremberg et al. [41] observed that a specific impedance was positively related with age until 13 years for both sexes, after which sex differences became apparent.

The assessment of BIVA patterns may assist in comparing adolescent athletes and identifying changes in body composition and the correlated hydration and cell mass qualitative information. BIVA identified the influence of age and strength in vector displacement. As the results show, handgrip strength may be an easier way to express biological maturity changes because of its correlation to FFM and how easy it is to be obtained. In fact, growth differences in female and male individuals are marked by the higher gain in FFM (and strength) in male than in female adolescents.

Handgrip strength is an acceptable indicator of overall muscle strength and health at any stage of life, from childhood to older age. BIVA is a promising alternative for assessing muscle strength, with potential application in other population groups.

5. Conclusions

The assessment of BIVA patterns may assist in comparing adolescent athletes and identifying changes in body composition and the correlated hydration and cell mass qualitative information. BIVA identified the influence of age and strength in vector displacement. As the results show, handgrip strength may be an easier way to express biological maturity changes, because of its correlation to FFM and how easy it is to be obtained. In fact, growth differences in female and male individuals are marked by the higher gain in FFM (and strength) in male than in female adolescents. Handgrip strength is an acceptable indicator of overall muscle strength and health at any stage of life, from childhood to older age. BIVA is a promising alternative for assessing muscle strength, with potential application in other population groups.

Author Contributions: Conceptualization, J.C.K. and M.V.d.O.C.; data curation, B.T.S.; formal analysis, M.V.d.O.C., F.C. and J.C.K.; investigation, J.C.K., M.V.d.O.C., F.C. and B.T.S.; writing—original draft preparation, J.C.K.; M.V.d.O.C.; B.T.S., F.C. and writing—review and editing, M.V.d.O.C., B.T.S., F.C. and J.C.K. All authors have read and agreed to the published version of the manuscript.

Funding: This research was funded by the Coordenação de Aperfeiçoamento de Nível Superior—Brasil (CAPES)—Finance code 001 and Fundação de Amparo à Pesquisa do Estado do Rio de Janeiro—(FAPERJ) E-26/010.001769/2019.

Institutional Review Board Statement: Protocols used in this study were approved by the Ethics Committee of Pedro Ernesto University Hospital (CEP/HUPE 649.202) and the Public Secretariat of Education (07/005.242/14). These protocols align with the Declaration of Helsinki of 1964.

Informed Consent Statement: Informed consent was obtained from all subjects involved in the study.

Acknowledgments: The authors thank all participants involved in this study and appreciate the collaboration of the school in carrying out the experiments, and Antonio Piccoli (Padua University, Italy) for kindly providing BIVA software (*in memorian*).

Conflicts of Interest: The authors declare no conflict of interest.

References

1. Rogol, A.D.; Clark, P.A.; Roemmich, J.N. Growth and pubertal development in children and adolescents: Effects of diet and physical activity. *Am. J. Clin. Nutr.* **2000**, *72*, 521S–528S. [CrossRef] [PubMed]
2. Bielemann, R.M.; Domingues, M.R.; Horta, B.L.; Menezes, A.M.B.; Gonçalves, H.; Assunção, M.C.F.; Hallal, P.C. Physical activity throughout adolescence and bone mineral density in early adulthood: The 1993 Pelotas (Brazil) Birth Cohort Study. *Osteoporos. Int.* **2014**, *25*, 2007–2015. [CrossRef]
3. Jiménez-Pavón, D.; Fernández-Vázquez, A.; Alexy, U.; Pedrero, R.; Cuenca-García, M.; Polito, A.; Vanhelst, J.; Manios, Y.; Kafatos, A.; Molnar, D.; et al. Association of objectively measured physical activity with body components in European adolescents. *BMC Public Health* **2013**, *13*, 667–675. [CrossRef]
4. Maughan, R.J.; Watson, J.S.; Weir, J. Strength and cross-sectional area of human skeletal muscle. *J. Physiol.* **1983**, *338*, 37–49. [CrossRef] [PubMed]
5. Moliner-Urdiales, D.; Ortega, F.B.; Vicente-Rodriguez, G.; Rey-Lopez, J.P.; Gracia-Marco, L.; Widhalm, K.; Sjöström, M.; Moreno, L.A.; Castillo, M.J.; Ruiz, J.R. Association of physical activity with muscular strength and fat-free mass in adolescents: The HELENA study. *Eur. J. Appl. Physiol.* **2010**, *109*, 1119–1127. [CrossRef]
6. Ubago-Guisado, E.; Vlachopoulos, D.; Ferreira de Moraes, A.C.; Torres-Costoso, A.; Wilkinson, K.; Metcalf, B.; Sánchez-Sánchez, J.; Gallardo, L.; Gracia-Marco, L. Lean mass explains the association between muscular fitness and bone outcomes in 13-year-old boys. *Acta Paediatr.* **2017**, *106*, 1658–1665. [CrossRef]
7. Campa, F.; Semprini, G.; Júdice, P.; Messina, G.; Toselli, S. Anthropometry, Physical and Movement Features, and Repeated-sprint Ability in Soccer Players. *Int. J. Sports Med.* **2019**, *40*, 100–109. [CrossRef] [PubMed]
8. Ortega, F.B.; Ruiz, J.R.; Castillo, M.J.; Sjöström, M. Physical fitness in childhood and adolescence: A powerful marker of health. *Int. J. Obes.* **2008**, *32*, 1–11. [CrossRef]
9. Richards, L.; Palmiter-Thomas, P. Grip strength measurement: A critical review of tools, methods, and clinical utility. *Crit. Rev. Phys. Rehabil. Med.* **1996**, *8*, 87–109. [CrossRef]
10. Silva, A.M. Structural and functional body components in athletic health and performance phenotypes. *Eur. J. Clin. Nutr.* **2019**, *73*, 215–224. [CrossRef]
11. Gómez-Campos, R.; Andruske, C.L.; de Arruda, M.; Sulla-Torres, J.; Pacheco-Carrillo, J.; Urra-Albornoz, C.; Cossio-Bolaños, M. Normative data for handgrip strength in children and adolescents in the Maule Region, Chile: Evaluation based on chronological and biological age. *PLoS ONE* **2018**, *13*, e0201033. [CrossRef]
12. Dugdale, J.H.; Arthur, C.A.; Sanders, D.; Hunter, A.M. Reliability and validity of field-based fitness tests in youth soccer players. *Eur. J. Sport Sci.* **2019**, *19*, 745–756. [CrossRef] [PubMed]
13. Pizzigalli, L.; Cremasco, M.M.; La Torre, A.; Rainoldi, A.; Benis, R. Hand grip strength and anthropometric characteristics in Italian female national basketball teams. *J. Sports Med. Phys. Fit.* **2017**, *57*, 521–528. [CrossRef]
14. Matias, C.N.; Santos, D.A.; Júdice, P.B.; Magalhães, J.P.; Minderico, C.S.; Fields, D.A.; Lukaski, H.C.; Sardinha, L.B.; Silva, A.M. Estimation of total body water and extracellular water with bioimpedance in athletes: A need for athlete-specific prediction models. *Clin. Nutr.* **2016**, *35*, 468–474. [CrossRef]
15. Moon, J.R. Body composition in athletes and sports nutrition: An examination of the bioimpedance analysis technique. *Eur. J. Clin. Nutr.* **2013**, *67*, S54–S59. [CrossRef]
16. Koury, J.C.; Ribeiro, M.A.; Massarani, F.A.; Vieira, F.; Marini, E. Fat-free mass in adolescent athletes: Accuracy of bioimpedance equations and identification of new predictive equations. *Nutrition* **2019**, *60*, 59–65. [CrossRef] [PubMed]
17. Castizo-Olier, J.; Irurtia, A.; Jemni, M.; Carrasco-Marginet, M.; Fernández-García, R.; Rodríguez, F.A. Bioelectrical impedance vector analysis (BIVA) in sport and exercise: Systematic review and future perspectives. *PLoS ONE* **2018**, *13*, e0197957. [CrossRef]
18. Marini, E.; Campa, F.; Buffa, R.; Stagi, S.; Matias, C.N.; Toselli, S.; Sardinha, L.B.; Silva, A.M. Phase angle and bioelectrical impedance vector analysis in the evaluation of body composition in athletes. *Clin. Nutr.* **2020**, *39*, 447–454. [CrossRef]
19. Piccoli, A.; Rossi, B.; Pillon, L.; Bucciante, G. A new method for monitoring body fluid variation by bioimpedance analysis: The RXc graph. *Kidney Int.* **1994**, *46*, 534–539. [CrossRef]
20. Baumgartner, R.N.; Chumlea, W.C.; Roche, A.F. Bioelectric impedance phase angle and body composition. *Am. J. Clin. Nutr.* **1988**, *48*, 16–23. [CrossRef] [PubMed]
21. Kyle, U.G.; Bosaeus, I.; De Lorenzo, A.D.; Deurenberg, P.; Elia, M.; Gómez, J.M.; Heitmann, B.L.; Kent-Smith, L.; Melchior, J.C.; Pirlich, M.; et al. Bioelectrical impedance analysis—Part II: Utilization in clinical practice. *Clin. Nutr.* **2004**, *23*, 1430–1453. [CrossRef]
22. Campa, F.; Matias, C.N.; Marini, E.; Heymsfield, S.B.; Toselli, S.; Sardinha, L.B.; Silva, A.M. Identifying Athlete Body Fluid Changes During a Competitive Season with Bioelectrical Impedance Vector Analysis. *Int. J. Sports Physiol. Perform.* **2020**, *15*, 361–367. [CrossRef] [PubMed]
23. Campa, F.; Matias, C.; Gatterer, H.; Toselli, S.; Koury, J.C.; Andreoli, A.; Melchiorri, G.; Sardinha, L.B.; Silva, A.M. Classic bioelectrical impedance vector reference values for assessing body composition in male and female athletes. *Int. J. Environ. Res. Public Health* **2019**, *16*, 5066. [CrossRef] [PubMed]
24. Desbrow, B.; Cox, G.; Desbrow, B.; Burke, L.M.; Cox, G.R.; Sawyer, S.M. Sports Dietitians Australia Position Statement: Sports Nutrition for the Adolescent Athlete Sports Dietitians Australia Position Statement: Sports Nutrition for the Adolescent Athlete. *Int. J. Sport Nutr. Exerc. Metab.* **2014**, *24*, 570–584. [CrossRef] [PubMed]

25. Malina, R.M.; Rogol, A.D.; Cumming, S.P.; Coelho e Silva, M.J.; Figueiredo, A.J. Biological maturation of youth athletes: Assessment and implications. *Br. J. Sports Med.* **2015**, *49*, 852–859. [CrossRef] [PubMed]
26. Mathias-Genovez, M.G.; Oliveira, C.C.; Camelo, J.S.; Del Ciampo, L.A.; Monteiro, J.P. Bioelectrical Impedance of Vectorial Analysis and Phase Angle in Adolescents. *J. Am. Coll. Nutr.* **2016**, *35*, 262–270. [CrossRef]
27. Horlick, M.; Arpadi, S.M.; Bethel, J.; Wang, J.; Moye, J.; Cuff, P.; Pierson, R.N.; Kotler, D. Bioelectrical impedance analysis models for prediction of total body water and fat-free mass in healthy and HIV-infected children and adolescents. *Am. J. Clin. Nutr.* **2002**, *76*, 991–999. [CrossRef]
28. Piccoli, A.; Pillon, L.; Dumler, F. Impedance vector distribution by sex, race, body mass index, and age in the United States: Standard reference intervals as bivariate Z scores. *Nutrition* **2002**, *18*, 153–167. [CrossRef]
29. Piccoli, A.; Pastori, G. *BIVA Software 2002*; Department of Medical and Surgical Sciences, University of Padova: Padova, Italy, 2002.
30. Ferreira, A.; Ara, D.; Batalha, N.; Collado-Mateo, D. Phase Angle from Bioelectric Impedance and Maturity-Related Factors in Adolescent Athletes: A Systematic Review. *Sustainability* **2020**, *12*, 4806–4820.
31. Koury, J.C.; Trugo, N.M.F.; Torres, A.G. Phase angle and bioelectrical impedance vectors in adolescent and adult male athletes. *Int. J. Sports Physiol. Perform.* **2014**, *9*, 798–804. [CrossRef]
32. Koury, J.C.; de Oliveira-Junior, A.V.; Portugal, M.R.C.; de Oliveira, K.d.J.F.; Donangelo, C.M. Bioimpedance parameters in adolescent athletes in relation to bone maturity and biochemical zinc indices. *J. Trace Elem. Med. Biol.* **2018**, *46*, 26–31. [CrossRef] [PubMed]
33. Dodds, R.M.; Syddall, H.E.; Cooper, R.; Kuh, D.; Cooper, C. Avan Aihie Sayer Global variation in grip strength: A systematic review and meta-analysis of normative data. *Age Ageing* **2016**, *45*, 209–216. [CrossRef] [PubMed]
34. De Palo, T.; Messina, G.; Edefonti, A.; Perfumo, F.; Pisanello, L.; Peruzzi, L.; Di Iorio, B.; Mignozzi, M.; Vienna, A.; Conti, G.; et al. Normal values of the bioelectrical impedance vector in childhood and puberty. *Nutrition* **2000**, *16*, 417–424. [CrossRef]
35. Toselli, S.; Marini, E.; Latessa, P.M.; Benedetti, L.; Campa, F. Maturity related differences in body composition assessed by classic and specific bioimpedance vector analysis among male elite youth soccer players. *Int. J. Environ. Res. Public Health* **2020**, *17*, 729. [CrossRef] [PubMed]
36. Rodríguez-Rodríguez, F.; Cristi-Montero, C.; González-Ruíz, K.; Correa-Bautista, J.E.; Ramírez-Vélez, R. Bioelectrical impedance vector analysis and muscular fitness in healthy men. *Nutrients* **2016**, *8*, 407. [CrossRef]
37. Mattiello, R.; Amaral, M.A.; Mundstock, E.; Ziegelmann, P.K. Reference values for the phase angle of the electrical bioimpedance: Systematic review and meta-analysis involving more than 250,000 subjects. *Clin. Nutr.* **2019**, *39*, 1411–1417. [CrossRef] [PubMed]
38. Campa, F.; Silva, A.M.; Iannuzzi, V.; Mascherini, G.; Benedetti, L.; Toselli, S. The role of somatic maturation on bioimpedance patterns and body composition in male elite youth soccer players. *Int. J. Environ. Res. Public Health* **2019**, *16*, 4711. [CrossRef]
39. Buffa, R.; Floris, G.; Marini, E. Bioelectrical impedance vector in pre- and postmenarcheal females. *Nutrition* **2002**, *18*, 474–478. [CrossRef]
40. Toselli, S.; Campa, F.; Latessa, P.M.; Greco, G.; Loi, A.; Grigoletto, A.; Zaccagni, L. Differences in maturity and anthropometric and morphological characteristics among young male basketball and soccer players and non-players. *Int. J. Environ. Res. Public Health* **2021**, *18*, 3902. [CrossRef]
41. Deurenberg, P.; Kusters, C.S.; Smit, H.E. Assessment of body composition by bioelectrical impedance in children and young adults is strongly age-dependent. *Eur. J. Clin. Nutr.* **1990**, *44*, 261–268.

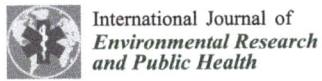

Article

Can Neurocognitive Function Predict Lower Extremity Injuries in Male Collegiate Athletes?

Sunghe Ha [1,2,†], Hee Seong Jeong [1,2,†], Sang-Kyoon Park [3,*,‡] and Sae Yong Lee [1,2,4,*,‡]

1. Department of Physical Education, College of Sciences in Education, Yonsei University, Seoul 03722, Korea; sunghe.ha@yonsei.ac.kr (S.H.); hsj@yonsei.ac.kr (H.S.J.)
2. International Olympic Committee Research Centre Korea, Yonsei University, Seoul 03722, Korea
3. School of Physical Education, Korea National Sport University, Seoul 05541, Korea
4. Institute of Convergence Science, Yonsei University, Seoul 03722, Korea
* Correspondence: spark@knsu.ac.kr (S.-K.P.); sylee1@yonsei.ac.kr (S.Y.L.);
  Tel.: +82-2-410-6952 (S.-K.P.); +82-2-2123-6189 (S.Y.L.); Fax: +82-2-410-6952 (S.-K.P.); +82-2-2123-8375 (S.Y.L.)
† The co-first authors (Sunghe Ha and Hee Seong Jeong) contributed equally to this work.
‡ The corresponding two authors (Sang-Kyoon Park and Sae Yong Lee) contributed equally to this work.

Received: 17 September 2020; Accepted: 2 December 2020; Published: 4 December 2020

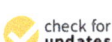

Abstract: The purpose of this study is to demonstrate whether neurocognitive evaluation can confirm the association between neurocognitive level and postural control and to analyze the relationship between neurocognitive level and acute musculoskeletal injury in male non-net sports athletes. Seventy-seven male non-net sports athletes participated in this study. The Standardized Assessment of Concussion (SAC), Landing Error Scoring System (LESS), Balance Error Scoring System (BESS), and Star Excursion Balance Test (SEBT) were used for testing; we collected data related to injury history for six months after testing. Pearson's correlation analysis, logistic regression, and the independent sample t-test were used for statistical analysis. The correlation between SAC and SEBT results was weak to moderate ($p < 0.05$). Eleven of the seventy-seven participants experienced acute lower limb injuries. SAC, LESS, BESS, and SEBT results have no effect on the occurrence of acute lower extremity injuries ($p > 0.05$) and were not statistically different between the injured and non-injured groups ($p > 0.05$). Therefore, using the SAC score alone to determine the risk factor of lower extremity injuries, except in the use of assessment after a concussion, should be cautioned against.

Keywords: lower limb; men; non-net sports; prevention; screening

1. Introduction

The occurrence of concussion among male elite athletes participating in contact sports is reported to be higher than that of women, accounting for approximately 66%–76% of the overall incidence [1–4]. In particular, the incidence of concussion was highest in adolescents and young adults [4]. Because of the nature of non-net sports such as contact with other players or objects, shocks to the head, neck, and upper body are frequent, and the accumulation of these shocks causes serious problems, for instance, concussions [5] and the possibility of cognitive decline [6]. According to a recent study analyzing the causal relationship between cognition and musculoskeletal injury, musculoskeletal injury may occur at a high level when participating in sports if the level of cognition is low or lowered owing to concussion [7–9]. Elite athletes who returned to sports after a concussion showed that the likelihood of acute lower musculoskeletal injury was increased compared with non-injured athletes [10,11].

Musculoskeletal injuries cause joint instability, recurrent injury, and other site injuries, as well as premature degenerative osteoarthritis [12] and accelerated retirement [13]. Various field studies have been reported to reduce the incidence of musculoskeletal injury, but several injuries have still been reported [14–16]. Along with current approaches to reduce sports injuries, new and efficient methods are needed in the field of sports. Most studies have suggested a link between cognition and sports injuries using expensive equipment such as computerized neurocognitive testing [17,18], magnetic response imaging [19], and electroencephalography [20]. However, a tool that can efficiently assess risk factors of musculoskeletal injury to athletes through a paper-and-pencil method and that is less expensive and requires less time than the computerized methods currently available is needed.

The Standardized Assessment of Concussion (SAC) was designed to quickly apply, observe, and evaluate the orientation, immediate memory, concentration, and delayed memory of an athlete with a head injury [21]. A reduction in SAC score according to head impact can be said to be a neurocognitive dysfunction [22]. Neurocognitive screening, the third item of the Sport Concussion Assessment Tool-Fifth Edition, is composed of SAC and is the most used method in the field [23,24]. However, its application as an assessment tool for neurocognitive impairment with regard to the accumulation of repetitive shocks during participation in non-net sports is insufficient. Repeated impact on the head results in decreased neurocognitive function, resulting in musculoskeletal injuries when participating in sports.

Due to the notion supported from neuroimage studies suggesting that the motor and neurocognitive process possesses the common neural pathway and resources [25–27], the studies trying to identify an association between neurocognitive function and postural control has been conducted [28,29]. This can explain the possibility of impairment of neuromuscular control if neurocognitive function has been damaged by repetitive impact. The association between neurocognitive function and motor skill may be affected by level of neurocognitive control process (difficulty/complexity of the task). Therefore, different types of field tasks assessing motor skills (e.g., static and dynamic postural control) should be employed to address and evaluate its association with neurocognitive function.

Static and dynamic balances are considered an important aspect of performance and injury risk of the lower extremity in many athletic events. Balance Error Scoring System (BESS), Landing Error Scoring System (LESS), Star Excursion Balance Test (SEBT), etc., used without expensive equipment in a clinical setting are applied to assess static and dynamic postural control capabilities, which are reported to be predictable for ligament sprains of the lower extremity [30–32]. These postural control test methods are not only used as baseline tests to monitor players before the season but also as evaluation criteria for returning to sports.

This study aims to verify whether neurocognitive assessment can identify association between neurocognitive level and postural control and analyze the association between the neurocognitive level and the occurrence of acute musculoskeletal injuries in male non-net sports athletes. This study hypothesized that there would be correlations between the neurocognitive evaluation scores and scores of postural control of the lower extremity, and the neurocognitive evaluation scores could predict acute lower limb injuries.

2. Methods

2.1. Participants

Seventy-seven male elite college players of 14 basketball, 22 rugby, 11 baseball, 15 ice hockey, and 15 soccer players participated in this study (height, 180.0 ± 7.4 cm; body weight, 83.9 ± 15.0 kg; age, 19.7 ± 1.3 y). All selected participants had no history of orthopedic acute injury or concussion in the previous six months, were registered as elite athletes, and participated in training and competition.

2.2. Experimental Design

This study was conducted with the approval of the Bioethics Committee of Yonsei University (7001988-201810-HR-465-03). Informed consent of voluntary participation was received from all study participants. After receiving informed consent, neurocognitive examination to detect injury risk of the lower extremity was performed using the screening tool, and follow-up investigation on injury occurrence was conducted.

2.2.1. Standardized Assessment of Concussion

As a noninvasive tool for determining brain dysfunction resulting from to sports concussion, the Korean version of SAC, which was verified for reliability and validity, was used for the neurocognitive evaluation test (conformity, 0.88–1.1; external compatibility, approximately 0.55–1.45; separation index, 4.59; separation reliability, 0.95) [33]. SAC is a form of scoring an answer through a tester's question and consists of a mental test, an immediate memory test, a concentration test (speaking in reverse order of numbers), a concentration test (subtracting 7 consecutive numbers from 100), and a delayed memory test. The total score for the Korean version is 37, with higher scores equating to better scores.

2.2.2. Postural Control of the Lower Extremity

Two video cameras (HDR-PJ410; Sony, Tokyo, Japan; EOS 800D; Canon, Tokyo, Japan) were used to evaluate the performance of the lower extremities (sampling rate, 60 Hz). Performing action is an evaluation tool for predicting lower limb injury and returning to rehabilitation. LESS, BESS, and SEBT have been used in the sports field.

In LESS, when the subject is ready for the motion test on a 30 cm box, the subject jumps both feet lightly and lands at 50% of the height and then immediately performs the maximum vertical jump (Figure 1A). A detailed explanation to perform the task successfully was provided to the participants and practice trials were provided three times. No feedback was provided during the task. If the instructions were followed, it was considered to be successful.

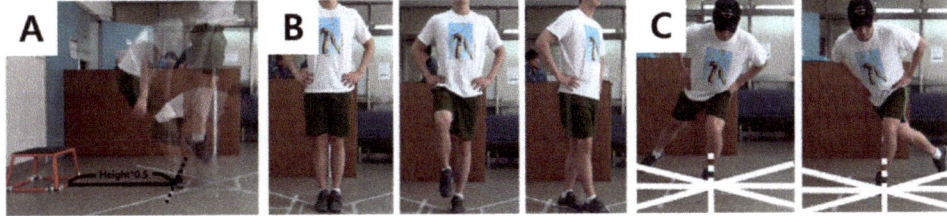

Figure 1. Experimental set-up to detect the injury risk of lower extremities: (**A**) Landing Error Scoring System; (**B**) Balance Error Scoring System; (**C**), Star Excursion Balance Test.

The BESS uses an action in which the subject closes his eyes and puts both hands on the right and left iliac crests and maintains double-leg standing (feet stand together), single-leg standing (on the nondominant leg), and tandem standing (nondominant foot behind the dominant foot) for 20 s each (Figure 1B). The ground condition was carried out on a flat floor and soft board. Participants were provided with a full description of the movement and warm-up, and practices were conducted thrice for each movement. No feedback was provided during the task.

In the SEBT (Figure 1C), the subjects stood on one leg in the center of the grid, with both hands placed on the left and right iliac crests. They were asked, along eight lines drawn at a 45-degree interval, to extend the legs as far as possible and touch the floor lightly with their toe. The direction of eight lines is as follows: anterior (A), anteromedial (AM), medial (M), posteromedial (PM), posterior (P), posterolateral (PL), lateral (L), and anterolateral (AL). If the subject falls off the fixed hand from the iliac crests and fails to stand on one foot or if the fixed footfalls or the foot fails to return to the starting position, it was considered a failure and was conducted again. Participants were provided with detailed instructions to successfully perform the task. A total of three practice tests were performed, and no feedback was provided during the task. The task was considered successful if the participants followed the instructions successfully.

For the follow-up of injury occurrence, the injury investigation form used by the International Olympic Committee was used for six months after neurocognitive examination and motion analysis [34]. The injury was defined as occurring acutely in the musculoskeletal system of the lower extremity, except for progressive onset and chronic pain. The history of injury of some participants who have team trainers was directly recorded by the trainer on the online-injury surveillance system, which was developed by YISSEM based on recommendations of International Olympic Committee, and was collected, and soccer participants without team trainers were contacted individually every two months by the author, with their injuries being recorded.

2.3. Data Processing

The SAC calculated the sub-domains and total score, respectively, for orientation, immediate memory, concentration, and delayed memory.

The LESS scored the error action by observing the initial contact of the ground, the maximum knee flexion, and the overall landing in the sagittal and coronal planes [30]. The lower the error score, the better the landing. The higher the score, the worse the landing (excellent landing, ≤4 points; good landing, 5 points; normal landing, 6 points; wrong landing, >6). There are 17 LESS items for error scoring: (1) the knee flexion angle of <30 degrees at initial contact (IC); (2) thigh in line with the trunk at IC; (3) trunk vertical or in line with the hips at IC; (4) foot landing heel to toe or with a flat foot at IC; (5) center of the patella being medial to the midfoot at IC; (6) trunk lateral flexion at IC; (7) asymmetric initial foot contact; (8) stance width greater than the shoulder width at IC; (9) stance width less than the shoulder width at IC; (10) external rotation of the foot >30 degrees between IC and maximum knee flexion; (11) internal rotation of the foot >30 degrees between IC and maximum knee flexion; (12) knee flexion angle of <45 degrees between IC and maximum knee flexion; (13) thigh not flexing more on the trunk between IC and maximum knee flexion; (14) trunk not flexing more between IC and maximum knee flexion; (15) center of the patella being medial to the great toe during landing; (16) displacement of the trunk, hips, and knees during landing; and (17) overall impression during landing [30]. Items 1–15 receive 1 point each if the above conditions are met. In contrast, item 16 is evaluated as 1 point for average and 2 points for stiff, and item 17 is evaluated as 1 point for average and 2 points for poor [30]. Kinovea (version 0.8.27; Kinovea, https://www.kinovea.org/) software was used to evaluate the knee angle among the items by the same rater (reliability: 0.941).

The BESS was conducted for 20 s. If an error of operation was observed 5 s before, 10 points were scored [35]. If an error was observed after 5 s, 1 point was added for each error operation, but if multiple errors occurred simultaneously, they were treated as 1 point [35]. The lower the error score, the better, and each action score and the total were calculated. There are five BESS items for error scoring: (1) raising the hand from the iliac crest; (2) opening your eyes; (3) any step, stumble, or fall; (4) the hip joint moved to over a 30-degree abduction; and (5) lifting the forefoot or heel [35]. The BESS results between repeat assessments by the same rater were excellent (reliability: 0.980).

The SEBT was calculated by standardizing the distance reached in each direction by the leg length (from the anterior iliac spine to the medial malleolus). The difference in reaching distance between both sides was the difference in distance from the dominant to the nondominant and was presented as an absolute value (Equation (1)) [31]. The length of the lower extremity and the distance to reach it were calculated by the same rater using the ratio method of Kinovea software (reliability: 0.917).

$$\text{Differences in reaching distance} = |Dominant\ leg - Nondominant\ leg| \qquad (1)$$

The incidence of injured musculoskeletal injuries in 77 participants collected over a 6-month period was calculated by frequency, type, and cause of injury and recovery period.

2.4. Statistical Analysis

Spearman's rank correlation analysis was performed for confirming the applicability of SAC to the evaluation tool for postural control of lower extremities. Binary logistic regression was performed to estimate the causal relationship between injury occurrence and SAC, injury occurrence, and postural control evaluation tools, respectively. An independent t-test and Mann–Whitney U-test were used to verify the difference in SAC score between the groups according to the presence or absence of lower limb damage and the postural control of the lower limb. SPSS 25.0 (IBM Corp., Armonk, NY, USA) was used for all statistical analysis, and the statistical significance level was set to $\alpha = 0.05$.

3. Results

3.1. The Correlation between SAC and Evaluation Tool for Postural Control of Lower Limb

Table 1 shows the correlation between the SAC score and the normalized reach distance of the SEBT's dominant and nondominant legs. A positive correlation was observed between the immediate memory score of SAC and the normalized reach distances of SEBT (P and PL of the dominant leg, and PM and P of the nondominant leg, respectively). A positive correlation was observed between the delayed memory and the normalized reach distance of the SEBT (PM, P, PL, and L of the dominant leg, and M, PM, P, and PL of the nondominant leg, respectively). Among the total scores of SAC and normalized P and PL reach the distance of SEBT of the dominant leg, a positive correlation was observed. The negative correlations were also observed between SAC (delayed memory and total score) and the M-direction difference between the dominant and nondominant legs (Table 2). On the other hand, no correlation was observed between SAC results compared with LESS, BESS, and SEBT results ($p > 0.05$).

Table 1. Correlation between neurocognitive testing score and normalized reaching distance in the Star Excursion Balance Test.

Items		A	AM	M	Dominant Leg PM	P	PL	L	AL
Orientation	ρ	0.127	0.126	0.077	−0.078	0.023	0.030	0.086	0.099
	p	0.269	0.277	0.505	0.502	0.845	0.797	0.459	0.391
Immediate memory	ρ	−0.058	0.169	0.125	0.210	0.341	0.359	0.216	0.018
	p	0.617	0.142	0.280	0.067	0.002 **	0.001 **	0.059	0.876
Concentration	ρ	−0.253	−0.120	−0.192	−0.101	0.017	−0.060	0.009	−0.193
	p	0.026	0.299	0.094	0.384	0.883	0.604	0.935	0.093
Delayed memory	ρ	−0.029	0.243	0.194	0.318	0.397	0.414	0.336	−0.023
	p	0.799	0.033	0.091	0.005 **	<0.001 ***	<0.001 ***	0.003 **	0.846
Total score	ρ	−0.155	0.083	0.007	0.127	0.301	0.247	0.209	−0.119
	p	0.178	0.472	0.951	0.272	0.008 **	0.030 *	0.068	0.302
					Nondominant Leg				
Orientation	ρ	0.037	0.004	−0.086	−0.069	−0.112	0.082	0.171	0.151
	p	0.750	0.971	0.459	0.549	0.332	0.480	0.137	0.189
Immediate memory	ρ	0.161	0.050	−0.163	0.312	0.316	0.194	0.106	0.010
	p	0.162	0.668	0.158	0.006 **	0.005 **	0.090	0.357	0.928
Concentration	ρ	−0.137	−0.224	−0.102	−0.149	−0.110	−0.159	−0.125	−0.035
	p	0.233	0.051	0.379	0.196	0.340	0.168	0.279	0.762
Delayed memory	ρ	0.164	0.072	0.243	0.374	0.338	0.225	0.113	0.078
	p	0.154	0.533	0.034 *	0.001 **	0.003 **	0.049 *	0.326	0.498
Total score	ρ	0.054	−0.077	0.099	0.161	0.177	0.065	0.016	−0.013
	p	0.644	0.505	0.392	0.163	0.124	0.573	0.893	0.909

A, anterior; AL, anterolateral; AM, anteromedial; L, lateral; M, medial; P, posterior; PL, posterolateral; PM, posteromedial. * $p < 0.05$; ** $p < 0.01$; *** $p < 0.001$.

Table 2. The correlation between neurocognitive testing score and differences of reaching distance in the Star Excursion Balance Test.

Domain		A	AM	M	PM	P	PL	L	AL
Orientation	ρ	0.075	−0.133	0.006	−0.213	0.086	−0.077	0.060	−0.137
	p	0.519	0.249	0.961	0.063	0.459	0.507	0.603	0.236
Immediate memory	ρ	−0.175	−0.023	−0.186	0.189	0.006	0.045	0.020	0.019
	p	0.128	0.841	0.105	0.099	0.962	0.694	0.864	0.869
Concentration	ρ	−0.081	−0.094	−0.215	−0.069	0.217	0.025	0.106	−0.130
	p	0.483	0.415	0.060	0.552	0.058	0.831	0.357	0.261
Delayed memory	ρ	−0.042	−0.001	−0.229	0.024	0.145	0.076	0.075	−0.138
	p	0.716	0.996	0.045 *	0.838	0.209	0.511	0.518	0.231
Total score	ρ	−0.150	−0.034	−0.253	0.050	0.199	0.054	0.123	−0.169
	p	0.194	0.770	0.027 *	0.669	0.083	0.640	0.287	0.143

A, anterior; AL, anterolateral; AM, anteromedial; L, lateral; M, medial; P, posterior; PL, posterolateral; PM, posteromedial. * $p < 0.05$.

3.2. Injury History for 6 Months after Testing

A total of 14 cases of acute musculoskeletal injury were reported in 77 participants collected over 6 months. Participants were classified into injured ($n = 11$) and healthy ($n = 66$) groups. One participant reported injuries to the ankle, lower leg, and hip, respectively, and the other participant reported injuries to the ankle and lower leg, respectively. The injured body parts were the ankle ($n = 5$, 35.7%), foot ($n = 1$, 7.1%), lower leg ($n = 2$, 14.3%), knee ($n = 2$, 14.3%), thigh ($n = 2$, 14.3%), and hip ($n = 2$, 14.3%). The types of injury included sprain ($n = 4$, 28.6%), strain ($n = 3$, 21.4%), bruise ($n = 3$, 21.4%), fracture ($n = 1$, 7.1%), ligament rupture ($n = 1$, 7.1%), cartilage injury ($n = 1$, 7.1%), and cramp ($n = 1$, 7.1%). The causes of injury were noncontact injury ($n = 9$, 64.3%), collision with other players ($n = 4$, 28.6%), and collision with moving objects ($n = 1$, 7.1%). The recovery period was 0 days ($n = 6$, 42.9%), 30 days or more ($n = 5$, 35.7%), 1 day ($n = 1$, 7.1%), 2 days ($n = 1$, 7.1%), and 7 days ($n = 1$, 7.1%).

3.3. Predicting Injury Occurrence

As a result of analyzing the accuracy of the classification of the injury occurrence group by logistic regression, the statistical significance of the individual independent variables for the presence or absence of injury was analyzed. Each result from logistic regression model suggests that the overall model was not found to be statistically significant ($p > 0.05$; Table 3). It was found that the independent variables (SAC, LESS, BESS, and SEBT) did not affect the presence or absence of injury ($p > 0.05$; Table 3).

Table 3. Final logistic regression results for the association of the variables with injuries.

Domain	β	p Value	OR	95% CI for OR
SAC				
Orientation	0.840	0.272	2.317	0.518 to 10.366
Immediate memory	0.273	0.502	1.314	0.592 to 2.920
Concentration	0.051	0.814	1.052	0.687 to 1.613
Delayed memory	0.305	0.426	1.356	0.641 to 2.871
Constant	−9.289	0.049	<0.001	
−2 Loglikelihood = 59.442, $\chi^2 = 5.083$ (df = 4, $p = 0.279$), Nagerkerke $R^2 = 0.114$				
LESS				
	−0.022	0.923	0.978	0.628 to 1.524
Constant	−1.694	0.110	0.184	
−2 Loglikelihood = 63.149, $\chi^2 = 0.009$ (df = 1, $p = 0.923$), Nagerkerke $R^2 < 0.001$				

Table 3. Cont.

Domain	β	p Value	OR	95% CI for OR
BESS				
Single-leg stance	−0.061	0.540	0.941	0.775 to 1.143
Tandem stance	−0.003	0.980	0.997	0.779 to 1.276
Double-leg stance on foam	0.392	0.219	1.480	0.792 to 2.766
Single-leg stance on foam	15.772	0.998	7,071,554.032	-
Tandem stance on foam	0.283	0.301	1.327	0.776 to 2.270
Constant	−161.821	0.998	<0.001	
−2 Loglikelihood = 57.640, χ^2 = 5.517 (df = 5, p = 0.356), Nagerkerke R^2 = 0.124				
Normalized reaching distance of dominant leg in SEBT				
Anterior	−0.023	0.690	0.977	0.871 to 1.096
Anteromedial	0.019	0.803	1.019	0.880 to 1.179
Medial	−0.018	0.492	0.982	0.934 to 1.033
Posteromedial	−0.049	0.293	0.952	0.869 to 1.043
Posterior	0.006	0.848	1.006	0.947 to 1.068
Posterolateral	0.079	0.098	1.082	0.985 to 1.189
Lateral	−0.020	0.652	0.980	0.898 to 1.070
Anterolateral	<0.001	0.997	1.000	0.934 to 1.071
Constant	−1.321	0.750	0.267	
−2 Loglikelihood = 59.442, χ^2 = 3.716 (df = 8, p = 0.882), Nagerkerke R^2 = 0.084				
Normalized reaching distance of nondominant leg in SEBT				
Anterior	0.002	0.966	1.002	0.897 to 1.120
Anteromedial	−0.021	0.752	0.979	0.860 to 1.115
Medial	−0.021	0.745	0.979	0.864 to 1.110
Posteromedial	0.034	0.484	1.035	0.940 to 1.139
Posterior	−0.009	0.839	0.991	0.906 to 1.083
Posterolateral	0.018	0.699	1.018	0.929 to 1.116
Lateral	−0.041	0.357	0.960	0.546 to 1.048
Anterolateral	0.031	0.540	1.031	0.935 to 1.138
Constant	−1.485	0.635	0.226	
−2 Loglikelihood = 61.393, χ^2 = 1.765 (df = 8, p = 0.987), Nagerkerke R^2 = 0.040				
Differences of reaching distance in SEBT				
Anterior	−0.014	0.879	0.986	0.826 to 1.178
Anteromedial	0.051	0.595	1.052	0.872 to 1.270
Medial	−0.073	0.407	0.930	0.783 to 1.104
Posteromedial	<0.001	0.998	1.000	0.870 to 1.149
Posterior	−0.040	0.558	0.961	0.842 to 1.097
Posterolateral	−0.003	0.963	0.997	0.873 to 1.138
Lateral	−0.107	0.235	0.898	0.753 to 1.072
Anterolateral	0.019	0.813	1.019	0.874 to 1.188
Constant	−0.821	0.455	0.440	
−2 Loglikelihood = 59.165, χ^2 = 3.993 (df = 8, p = 0.858), Nagerkerke R^2 = 0.090				

BESS, Balance Error Scoring System; CI, confidence interval; df, degree of freedom; LESS, Landing Error Scoring System; OR, odds ratio; SAC, Standardized Assessment of Concussion; SEBT, Star Excursion Balance Test.

3.4. Difference between Injured and Healthy Groups

Statistical differences between groups were not observed in the SAC score and lower limb function performance evaluation results (Table 4).

Table 4. The results of the independent *t*-test between non-injured and injured groups.

Domain	Non-Injured (n = 66)	Injured (n = 11)	Z t (df) §	p Value
SAC				
Orientation	4.53 ± 0.56	4.73 ± 0.47	1.074	0.283
Immediate memory	5.70 ± 1.21	6.27 ± 1.19	1.441	0.150
Concentration	7.89 ± 1.70	8.27 ± 1.27	0.550	0.583
Delayed memory	4.70 ± 1.14	5.45 ± 1.57	1.524	0.127
Total score	22.82 ± 3.05	24.73 ± 3.07	1.923 (75) §	0.058
LESS				
Total error of LESS	4.50 ± 1.38	4.45 ± 1.86	0.447	0.655
BESS				
Double-leg stance	0.00 ± 0.00	0.00 ± 0.00		
Single-leg stance	6.53 ± 3.50	6.00 ± 3.46	−0.536	0.592
Tandem stance	2.29 ± 2.68	2.73 ± 3.00	0.657	0.511
Double-leg stance on foam	0.23 ± 0.65	0.64 ± 1.43	0.586	0.558
Single-leg stance on foam	9.70 ±1.35	10.00 ± 0.00	1.034	0.301
Tandem stance on foam	8.67 ± 2.45	9.64 ± 0.92	0.956	0.339
Total error of BESS	27.41 ± 6.25	29.00 ± 5.78	0.789 (75) §	0.433
Normalized reaching distance of dominant leg in SEBT				
Anterior	80.77 ± 10.35	79.05 ± 6.42	0.533 (75) §	0.596
Anteromedial	86.65 ± 12.28	85.39 ± 6.48	0.262	0.793
Medial	88.20 ± 15.64	85.95 ± 8.36	−0.742	0.458
Posteromedial	94.66 ± 13.91	93.28 ± 10.14	0.316 (75) §	0.753
Posterior	86.90 ± 14.29	88.14 ± 7.16	−0.282 (75) §	0.779
Posterolateral	86.09 ± 14.51	89.73 ± 8.99	1.121	0.262
Lateral	75.30 ± 15.23	76.34 ± 8.26	<0.001	1.000
Anterolateral	72.68 ± 12.93	72.60 ± 11.28	0.020 (75) §	0.984
Normalized reaching distance of nondominant leg in SEBT				
Anterior	80.94 ± 11.48	80.42 ± 6.85	0.102	0.919
Anteromedial	88.37 ± 11.77	86.80 ± 8.04	0.425 (75) §	0.672
Medial	90.10 ± 12.29	88.94 ± 7.59	−0.480	0.631
Posteromedial	96.45 ± 14.76	97.12 ± 11.51	0.269	0.788
Posterior	88.24 ± 14.90	87.29 ± 6.21	0.335	0.738
Posterolateral	83.43 ± 14.18	83.37 ± 6.02	0.015 (75) §	0.988
Lateral	73.99 ± 14.31	71.53 ± 8.54	0.552 (75) §	0.582
Anterolateral	71.05 ± 11.46	71.15 ± 8.54	−0.027 (75) §	0.978
Differences of reaching distance in SEBT				
Anterior	4.70 ± 3.95	4.12 ± 3.86	−0.655	0.512
Anteromedial	4.83 ± 3.85	5.41 ± 4.48	0.291	0.771
Medial	7.52 ± 10.70	5.40 ± 3.33	−0.524	0.600
Posteromedial	6.40 ± 5.58	6.53 ± 4.12	0.590	0.555
Posterior	6.06 ± 9.80	4.54 ± 2.90	0.029	0.977
Posterolateral	7.53 ± 6.04	6.87 ± 5.43	−0.175	0.861
Lateral	6.87 ± 5.00	4.73 ± 3.71	−1.310	0.190
Anterolateral	5.19 ± 4.76	6.68 ± 2.77	1.791	0.073

BESS, Balance Error Scoring System; df, degree of freedom; LESS, Landing Error Scoring System; M, mean; SAC, Standardized Assessment of Concussion; SD, standard deviation; SEBT, Star Excursion Balance Test; §, Independent *t*-test value. Values are expressed as mean ± standard deviation.

4. Discussion

This study aims to assess if neurocognitive assessment can identify risk factors of the lower extremity and to analyze the association between the neurocognitive level and the occurrence of acute musculoskeletal injuries in male collegiate athletes. The major findings of this study are twofold: first, SAC evaluating neurocognitive function of collegiate athletes and dynamic postural control have small to medium correlations, and second, however, lower extremity injuries cannot be predicted using the SAC. As a result of this study, the correlation between SAC results (immediate memory, delayed memory, and total score) and SEBT result was observed. This result was consistent with our hypothesis. Even though motor skills including gross control such as balance, walking, agility, and flexibility were weakly associated with neurocognitive skills, neurocognitive function has been reported to be associated with motor skills, which may support the result of this study. The strength of link between neurocognitive function and motor skill is influenced by the difficulty of the task [36–38]. Therefore, SEBT, which is dynamic postural assessment tool, can be a difficult motor skill (novelty, complex/difficult task) that can be affected by neurocognitive function [25,39–41]. Since SEBT is more goal directed motor action and need specific (high-order) neurocognitive control process, SEBT is more likely to be affected by neurocognitive level than other balance task. According to the results of a prospective cohort using SEBT, lower limb injuries were reported in high school basketball players with normalized A, PM, and PL reach of 94% or less [31]. In addition, a systematic review has reported that SEBT is associated with an increased risk of injury [42,43]. This study suggests the possibility of predicting lower extremity injuries through correlation between the memory area that is the sub-domain of the SAC and SEBT result.

Based on the results of this study, it was found that lower extremity injuries cannot be predicted using the SAC. This result was inconsistent with our hypothesis. In a study conducted on alpine skiers and snowboarders, there was no difference in neurocognitive scores between the injured and non-injured groups, which is similar to the results of the present study [44]. Although the neurocognitive evaluation was applied to those who did not have a history of concussion within the past six months when recruiting the participants, it is thought that the cumulative shock received by the subjects participating in each of their sports during the six months of data collection may have resulted in impairment that may have affected neurocognitive function. These effects would have decreased physical function and increased the risk of musculoskeletal injury and concussion [45]. Therefore, it is necessary to periodically record and observe SAC scores for athletes who participate in non-net sports.

The criteria for judging sports concussion during training and competition are classified by coaching staff in the field according to the athlete's awareness and loss of consciousness. The understanding of both players and leaders regarding concussion was high, but there was a problem with the classification and management of the actual concussion [46,47]. The recovery period of a simple concussion is reported to occur immediately or within 10 days, depending on the degree [48,49]. However, some athletes do not fully recover from concussion and are more likely to be exposed to other injuries when returning to the field [11,50]. Athletes are reluctant to talk about their symptoms because of the fear of being excluded from the entry list. In the case of the subjects of this study, it is possible that less number of injuries was reported to the team trainer because they are selected to the professional team based on their grades on the university team.

In the SAC results of this study, no statistical difference was observed between the injured and non-injured groups. Ha reported that have no difference in scores of computerized neurocognitive tests between retired contact-sports athletes and control [51]. However, retired contact-sports athletes showed slower gait speeds during dual-task walking because the cognitive task is preceded any movement for walking [51]. A decline in neurocognitive ability may reduce the ability to cope with rapidly changing situations and increase the likelihood of injury. Previous studies have reported that cardiopulmonary training [52] and resistance training [53] improve memory and selective concentration, which are sub-domains of neurocognitive ability. Although athletes who participate in non-net sports repeatedly experience impacts on the head, it is thought that aerobic training and resistance training, in which the athletes regularly participated to improve physical ability, also influenced neurocognitive ability. Therefore, there might be difficulties in predicting injury through changes in neurocognition while participating in sports competitions and training. However, loss of proprioception information due to a past history of musculoskeletal injury and reduction in sports activities after retirements, such as understanding tactics and aerobic exercise, can cause a decrease in neurocognitive ability.

Nevertheless, this study has some limitations. First, the injury follow-up period was as short as six months. A previous study reported that 6–12 months after concussion were greater incidence of the lower extremity injury than 0 to 3 and 3 to 6 months [11]. In future studies, the duration of injury follow-up should be considered. Second, the injured group that was investigated had a relatively small sample size, which is a usual limitation in prospective research. Therefore, further research is needed because the resulting analysis is subject to limitations. Third, baseball and basketball, which have relatively low concussion rates, were included in this study. However, traumatic brain injury has been an important issue in baseball [54]. Some concussed baseball players showed no symptoms when they returned to play, but residual effects on their batting technique were reported [55]. Cognition and perception are the most important factors in playing basketball [56]. If a head injury such as a concussion occurs, these can be affected. Unfortunately, basketball had the highest competition-related rates of concussion for partial-contact sports such as soccer [57]. Fourth, the SAC has so far been used as a cognitive evaluation tool in sports sites [23], but this method was designed about twenty years ago. Because there is a point of contention in the method, which was developed some time ago, further research will be required for the development of a new cognitive evaluation tool that is both valid and reliable. Lastly, follow-up data about the injury incidence were not collected in the same way because the trainer's employment was different, which depended on the participants' team circumstances.

5. Conclusions

The SAC score of college male non-net sports players alone was unable to predict the occurrence of injury. Therefore, using the SAC score alone to determine the risk factor of lower extremity injuries, except in the use of assessment after a concussion, should be cautioned against.

Author Contributions: Study design, S.H., H.S.J., S.-K.P., and S.Y.L.; study conduct, S.H., H.S.J., S.-K.P., and S.Y.L.; data collection, S.H., and H.S.J.; data analysis, S.H., and H.S.J.; data interpretation, S.H., H.S.J., S.-K.P., and S.Y.L.; drafting manuscript, S.H., H.S.J. and S.Y.L.; revising manuscript content, S.H., H.S.J., S.-K.P., and S.Y.L. All authors have read and agreed to the published version of the manuscript.

Funding: This work was supported by the Ministry of Education of the Republic of Korea and the National Research Foundation of Korea (NRF-2018S1A5B5A01032989).

Acknowledgments: The authors would like to thank all of the participants, as well as Jae Ho Kim and Kun Wang, for their help in collecting the data.

Conflicts of Interest: The authors declare no conflict of interest.

References

1. Theadom, A.; Starkey, N.J.; Dowell, T.; Hume, P.A.; Kahan, M.; McPherson, K.; Feigin, V.; BIONIC Research Group. Sports-related brain injury in the general population: An epidemiological study. *J. Sci. Med. Sport* **2014**, *17*, 591–596. [CrossRef] [PubMed]
2. Ingebrigtsen, T.; Waterloo, K.; Marup-Jensen, S.; Attner, E.; Romner, B. Quantification of post-concussion symptoms 3 months after minor head injury in 100 consecutive patients. *J. Neurol.* **1998**, *245*, 609–612. [CrossRef] [PubMed]
3. Servadei, F.; Verlicchi, A.; Soldano, F.; Zanotti, B.; Piffer, S. Descriptive epidemiology of head injury in Romagna and Trentino. Comparison between two geographically different Italian regions. *Neuroepidemiology* **2002**, *21*, 297–304. [CrossRef] [PubMed]
4. Theadom, A.; Mahon, S.; Hume, P.; Starkey, N.; Barker-Collo, S.; Jones, K.; Majdan, M.; Feigin, V.L. Incidence of sports-related traumatic brain injury of all severities: A systematic review. *Neuroepidemiology* **2020**, *54*, 192–199. [CrossRef] [PubMed]
5. King, D.; Hume, P.; Gissane, C.; Brughelli, M.; Clark, T. The influence of head impact threshold for reporting data in contact and collision sports: Systematic review and original data analysis. *Sports Med.* **2016**, *46*, 151–169. [CrossRef]

6. Kim, G.H.; Kang, I.; Jeong, H.; Park, S.; Hong, H.; Kim, J.; Kim, J.Y.; Edden, R.A.E.; Lyoo, I.K.; Yoon, S. Low prefrontal GABA levels are associated with poor cognitive functions in professional boxers. *Front. Hum. Neurosci.* **2019**, *13*, 193. [CrossRef]
7. Herman, D.C.; Zaremski, J.L.; Vincent, H.K.; Vincent, K.R. Effect of neurocognition and concussion on musculoskeletal injury risk. *Curr. Sports Med. Rep.* **2015**, *14*, 194–199. [CrossRef]
8. Swanik, C.B. Brains and sprains: The brain's role in noncontact anterior cruciate ligament injuries. *J. Athl. Train.* **2015**, *50*, 1100–1102. [CrossRef]
9. Wilkerson, G.B. Neurocognitive reaction time predicts lower extremity sprains and strains. *Int. J. Athl. Ther. Train.* **2012**, *17*, 4–9. [CrossRef]
10. Brooks, M.A.; Peterson, K.; Biese, K.; Sanfilippo, J.; Heiderscheit, B.C.; Bell, D.R. Concussion increases odds of sustaining a lower extremity musculoskeletal injury after return to play among collegiate athletes. *Am. J. Sports Med.* **2016**, *44*, 742–747. [CrossRef]
11. Nordstrom, A.; Nordstrom, P.; Ekstrand, J. Sports-related concussion increases the risk of subsequent injury by about 50% in elite male football players. *Br. J. Sports Med.* **2014**, *48*, 1447–1450. [CrossRef] [PubMed]
12. Lohmander, L.S.; Ostenberg, A.; Englund, M.; Roos, H. High prevalence of knee osteoarthritis, pain, and functional limitations in female soccer players twelve years after anterior cruciate ligament injury. *Arthritis Rheum.* **2004**, *50*, 3145–3152. [CrossRef] [PubMed]
13. Secrist, E.S.; Bhat, S.B.; Dodson, C.C. The financial and professional impact of anterior cruciate ligament injuries in National Football League athletes. *Orthop. J. Sports Med.* **2016**, *4*, 2325967116663921. [CrossRef] [PubMed]
14. Hewett, T.E.; Myer, G.D.; Ford, K.R.; Paterno, M.V.; Quatman, C.E. Mechanisms, prediction, and prevention of ACL injuries: Cut risk with three sharpened and validated tools. *J. Orthop. Res.* **2016**, *34*, 1843–1855. [CrossRef] [PubMed]
15. Gledhill, A.; Forsdyke, D. An ounce of prevention is better than a pound of cure: Shouldn't we be doing EVERYTHING to reduce sports injury incidence and burden? *Br. J. Sports Med.* **2018**, *52*, 1292–1293. [CrossRef] [PubMed]
16. Jacobsson, J.; Timpka, T. Classification of prevention in sports medicine and epidemiology. *Sports Med.* **2015**, *45*, 1483–1487. [CrossRef]
17. Hutchison, M.; Comper, P.; Mainwaring, L.; Richards, D. The influence of musculoskeletal injury on cognition: Implications for concussion research. *Am. J. Sports Med.* **2011**, *39*, 2331–2337. [CrossRef]
18. Swanik, C.B.; Covassin, T.; Stearne, D.J.; Schatz, P. The relationship between neurocognitive function and noncontact anterior cruciate ligament injuries. *Am. J. Sports Med.* **2007**, *35*, 943–948. [CrossRef]
19. Kapreli, E.; Athanasopoulos, S.; Gliatis, J.; Papathanasiou, M.; Peeters, R.; Strimpakos, N.; Hecke, P.V.; Gouliamos, A.; Sunaert, S. Anterior cruciate ligament deficiency causes brain plasticity: A functional MRI study. *Am. J. Sports Med.* **2009**, *37*, 2419–2426. [CrossRef]
20. Bonnette, S.; Diekfuss, J.A.; Grooms, D.R.; Kiefer, A.W.; Riley, M.A.; Riehm, C.; Moore, C.; Foss, K.D.B.; DiCesare, C.A.; Baumeister, J.; et al. Electrocortical dynamics differentiate athletes exhibiting low-and high-ACL injury risk biomechanics. *Psychophysiology* **2020**, *57*, e13530. [CrossRef]
21. McCrea, M. Standardized mental status testing on the sideline after sport-related concussion. *J. Athl. Train.* **2001**, *36*, 274–279.
22. Dessy, A.M.; Yuk, F.J.; Maniya, A.Y.; Gometz, A.; Rasouli, J.J.; Lovell, M.R.; Choudhri, T.F. Review of assessment scales for diagnosing and monitoring sports-related concussion. *Cureus* **2017**, *9*, e1922. [CrossRef] [PubMed]
23. Echemendia, R.J.; Meeuwisse, W.; McCrory, P.; Davis, G.A.; Putukian, M.; Leddy, J.; Makdissi, M.; Sullivan, S.J.; Broglio, S.P.; Raftery, M.; et al. The sport concussion assessment tool 5th edition (SCAT5): Background and rationale. *Br. J. Sports Med.* **2017**, *51*, 848–850. [PubMed]
24. Murphy, A.; Kaufman, M.S.; Molton, I.; Coppel, D.B.; Benson, J.; Herring, S.A. Concussion evaluation methods among Washington State high school football coaches and athletic trainers. *PM&R* **2012**, *4*, 419–426.
25. Diamond, A. Close interrelation of motor development and cognitive development and of the cerebellum and prefrontal cortex. *Child Dev.* **2000**, *71*, 44–56. [CrossRef] [PubMed]
26. Serrien, D.J.; Ivry, R.B.; Swinnen, S.P. Dynamics of hemispheric specialization and integration in the context of motor control. *Nat. Rev. Neurosci.* **2006**, *7*, 160–166. [CrossRef]

27. Fuelscher, I.; Caeyenberghs, K.; Enticott, P.G.; Williams, J.; Lum, J.; Hyde, C. Differential activation of brain areas in children with developmental coordination disorder during tasks of manual dexterity: An ALE meta-analysis. *Neurosci. Biobehav. Rev.* **2018**, *86*, 77–84. [CrossRef]
28. Alsalaheen, B.A.; Whitney, S.L.; Marchetti, G.F.; Furman, J.M.; Kontos, A.P.; Collins, M.W.; Sparto, P.J. Relationship between cognitive assessment and balance measures in adolescents referred for vestibular physical therapy after concussion. *Clin. J. Sport Med.* **2016**, *26*, 46–52. [CrossRef]
29. Parker, T.M.; Osternig, L.R.; van Donkelaar, P.; Chou, L.S. Recovery of cognitive and dynamic motor function following concussion. *Br. J. Sports Med.* **2007**, *41*, 868–873. [CrossRef]
30. Padua, D.A.; Marshall, S.W.; Boling, M.C.; Thigpen, C.A.; Garrett Jr, W.E.; Beutler, A.I. The Landing Error Scoring System (LESS) is a valid and reliable clinical assessment tool of jump-landing biomechanics: The JUMP-ACL study. *Am. J. Sports Med.* **2009**, *37*, 1996–2002. [CrossRef]
31. Plisky, P.J.; Rauh, M.J.; Kaminski, T.W.; Underwood, F.B. Star Excursion Balance Test as a predictor of lower extremity injury in high school basketball players. *J. Orthop. Sports Phys. Ther.* **2006**, *36*, 911–919. [CrossRef] [PubMed]
32. McGuine, T.A.; Greene, J.J.; Best, T.; Leverson, G. Balance as a predictor of ankle injuries in high school basketball players. *Clin. J. Sport Med.* **2000**, *10*, 239–244. [CrossRef] [PubMed]
33. Mun, J. Developement of a Concussion Assessment Instrument for the South Korean Soldiers. Ph.D. Thesis, Middle Tennessee State University, Murfreesboro, TN, USA, December 2017.
34. Junge, A.; Engebretsen, L.; Alonso, J.M.; Renstrom, P.; Mountjoy, M.L.; Aubry, M.; Dvorak, J. Injury surveillance in multi-sport events: The International Olympic Committee approach. *Br. J. Sports Med.* **2008**, *42*, 413–421. [CrossRef]
35. Starling, A.J.; Leong, D.F.; Bogle, J.M.; Vargas, B.B. Variability of the modified Balance Error Scoring System at baseline using objective and subjective balance measures. *Concussion* **2016**, *1*, CNC5. [CrossRef] [PubMed]
36. Stuhr, C.; Hughes, C.M.L.; Stöckel, T. Task-specific and variability-driven activation of cognitive control processes during motor performance. *Sci. Rep.* **2018**, *8*, 10811. [CrossRef]
37. Norouzi, E.; Vaezmosavi, M.; Gerber, M.; Pühse, U.; Brand, S. Dual-task training on cognition and resistance training improved both balance and working memory in older people. *Phys. Sportsmed.* **2019**, *47*, 471–478. [CrossRef]
38. Geertsen, S.S.; Thomas, R.; Larsen, M.N.; Dahn, I.M.; Andersen, J.N.; Krause-Jensen, M.; Korup, V.; Nielsen, C.M.; Wienecke, J.; Ritz, C. Motor skills and exercise capacity are associated with objective measures of cognitive functions and academic performance in preadolescent children. *PLoS ONE* **2016**, *11*, e0161960. [CrossRef]
39. Diamond, A. Activities and programs that improve children's executive functions. *Curr. Dir. Psychol. Sci.* **2012**, *21*, 335–341. [CrossRef]
40. Espy, K.A.; McDiarmid, M.M.; Cwik, M.F.; Stalets, M.M.; Hamby, A.; Senn, T.E. The contribution of executive functions to emergent mathematic skills in preschool children. *Dev. Neuropsychol.* **2004**, *26*, 465–486. [CrossRef] [PubMed]
41. Poldrack, R.A.; Sabb, F.W.; Foerde, K.; Tom, S.M.; Asarnow, R.F.; Bookheimer, S.Y.; Knowlton, B.J. The neural correlates of motor skill automaticity. *J. Neurosci.* **2005**, *25*, 5356–5364. [CrossRef]
42. Hegedus, E.J.; McDonough, S.M.; Bleakley, C.; Baxter, D.; Cook, C.E. Clinician-friendly lower extremity physical performance tests in athletes: A systematic review of measurement properties and correlation with injury. Part 2—The tests for the hip, thigh, foot and ankle including the star excursion balance test. *Br. J. Sports Med.* **2015**, *49*, 649–656. [CrossRef] [PubMed]
43. Gribble, P.A.; Hertel, J.; Plisky, P. Using the Star Excursion Balance Test to assess dynamic postural-control deficits and outcomes in lower extremity injury: A literature and systematic review. *J. Athl. Train.* **2012**, *47*, 339–357. [CrossRef] [PubMed]
44. Faltus, J.; Huntimer, B.; Kernozek, T.; Cole, J. Utilization of ImPACT testing to measure injury risk in Alpine ski and Snowboard athletes. *Int. J. Sports Phys. Ther.* **2016**, *11*, 498–506. [PubMed]
45. Herman, D.C.; Barth, J.T. Drop-jump landing varies with baseline neurocognition: Implications for anterior cruciate ligament injury risk and prevention. *Am. J. Sports Med.* **2016**, *44*, 2347–2353. [CrossRef] [PubMed]
46. Kirk, B.; Pugh, J.N.; Cousins, R.; Phillips, S.M. Concussion in university level sport: Knowledge and awareness of athletes and coaches. *Sports* **2018**, *6*, 102. [CrossRef]

47. O'Connell, E.; Molloy, M.G. Concussion in rugby: Knowledge and attitudes of players. *Ir. J. Med. Sci.* **2016**, *185*, 521–528. [CrossRef]
48. Macciocchi, S.N.; Barth, J.T.; Alves, W.; Rimel, R.W.; Jane, J.A. Neuropsychological functioning and recovery after mild head injury in collegiate athletes. *Neurosurgery* **1996**, *39*, 510–514. [CrossRef]
49. Maroon, J.C.; Lovell, M.R.; Norwig, J.; Podell, K.; Powell, J.W.; Hartl, R. Cerebral concussion in athletes: Evaluation and neuropsychological testing. *Neurosurgery* **2000**, *47*, 659–672.
50. Kim, S.; Han, D.; Lee, J. Prevalence and correlates of impairments in activities of daily living in older Koreans: Comparison of young-old and old-old. *J. Mens Health* **2019**, *15*, e1–e10. [CrossRef]
51. Ha, S. Effects of participation in contact sports on neurocognitive scores and dual-task walking in retired athletes. *KJSB* **2020**, *30*, 265–273.
52. Thomas, A.G.; Dennis, A.; Rawlings, N.B.; Stagg, C.J.; Matthews, L.; Morrisc, M.; Kolind, S.H.; Foxley, S.; Jenkinson, M.; Nichols, T.E.; et al. Multi-modal characterization of rapid anterior hippocampal volume increase associated with aerobic exercise. *Neuroimage* **2016**, *131*, 162–170. [CrossRef] [PubMed]
53. Liu-Ambrose, T.; Nagamatsu, L.S.; Voss, M.W.; Khan, K.M.; Handy, T.C. Resistance training and functional plasticity of the aging brain: A 12-month randomized controlled trial. *Neurobiol. Aging* **2012**, *33*, 1690–1698. [CrossRef] [PubMed]
54. Green, G.A.; Pollack, K.M.; D'Angelo, J.; Schickendantz, M.S.; Caplinger, R.; Weber, K.; Valadka, A.; McAllister, T.W.; Dick, R.W.; Mandelbaum, B.; et al. Mild traumatic brain injury in Major and Minor League Baseball players. *Am. J. Sports Med.* **2015**, *43*, 1118–1126. [CrossRef] [PubMed]
55. Wasserman, E.B.; Abar, B.; Shah, M.N.; Wasserman, D.; Bazarian, J.J. Concussions are associated with decreased batting performance among Major League Baseball players. *Am. J. Sports Med.* **2015**, *43*, 1127–1133. [CrossRef]
56. Kioumourtzoglou, E.; Derri, V.; Tzetzls, G.; Theodorakis, Y. Cognitive, perceptual, and motor abilities in skilled basketball performance. *Percept. Mot. Skills* **1998**, *86*, 771–786. [CrossRef]
57. Gessel, L.M.; Fields, S.K.; Collins, C.L.; Dick, R.W.; Comstock, R.D. Concussions among United States high school and collegiate athletes. *J. Athl. Train.* **2007**, *42*, 495–503.

Publisher's Note: MDPI stays neutral with regard to jurisdictional claims in published maps and institutional affiliations.

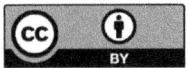

© 2020 by the authors. Licensee MDPI, Basel, Switzerland. This article is an open access article distributed under the terms and conditions of the Creative Commons Attribution (CC BY) license (http://creativecommons.org/licenses/by/4.0/).

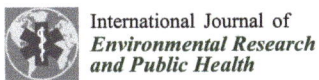

Review

The Effects of Resistance Training on Blood Pressure in Preadolescents and Adolescents: A Systematic Review and Meta-Analysis

Carles Miguel Guillem [1], Andrés Felipe Loaiza-Betancur [2], Tamara Rial Rebullido [3], Avery D. Faigenbaum [4] and Iván Chulvi-Medrano [5,*]

1. Department of Physical and Sports Education, Faculty of Physical Activity and Sport Sciences, University of Valencia, 46010 Valencia, Spain; carlesmg7@gmail.com
2. University Institute of Physical Education, University of Antioquia, Medellín 1226, Colombia; andres.loaiza@udea.edu.co
3. Tamara Rial Exercise & Women's Health, Newtown, PA 18940, USA; rialtamara@gmail.com
4. Department of Health and Exercise Science, The College of New Jersey, Ewing, NJ 08628, USA; faigenba@tcnj.edu
5. UIRFIDE (Sport Performance and Physical Fitness Research Group), Department of Physical and Sports Education, Faculty of Physical Activity and Sports Sciences, University of Valencia, 46010 Valencia, Spain
* Correspondence: ivan.chulvi@uv.es

Received: 27 September 2020; Accepted: 23 October 2020; Published: 28 October 2020

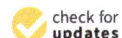

Abstract: The aim was to systematically review and meta-analyze the current evidence for the effects of resistance training (RT) on blood pressure (BP) as the main outcome and body mass index (BMI) in children and adolescents. Two authors systematically searched the PubMed, SPORTDiscus, Web of Science Core Collection and EMBASE electronic databases. Inclusion criteria were: (1) children and adolescents (aged 8 to 18 years); (2) intervention studies including RT and (3) outcome measures of BP and BMI. The selected studies were analyzed using the Cochrane Risk-of-Bias Tool. Eight articles met inclusion criteria totaling 571 participants. The mean age ranged from 9.3 to 15.9 years and the mean BMI of 29.34 (7.24) kg/m^2). Meta-analysis indicated that RT reduced BMI significantly (mean difference (MD): −0.43 kg/m^2 (95% CI: −0.82, −0.03), P = 0.03; I^2 = 5%) and a non-significant decrease in systolic BP (SBP) (MD: −1.09 mmHg (95% CI: −3.24, 1.07), P = 0.32; I^2 = 67%) and diastolic BP (DBP) (MD: −0.93 mmHg (95% CI: −2.05, 0.19), P = 0.10; I^2 = 37%). Limited evidence suggests that RT has no adverse effects on BP and may positively affect BP in youths. More high-quality studies are needed to clarify the association between RT and BP in light of body composition changes throughout childhood and adolescence.

Keywords: children; youths; neuromuscular training; cardiovascular health; overweight; obesity

1. Introduction

The treatment for hypertension is usually pharmacological and has shown to be effective in 50% of adult patients [1]. However, in younger populations pharmacological treatment should be reserved for those who present with persistent elevated blood pressure (BP) despite lifestyle modification [2]. Therefore, it is reasonable to investigate non-pharmacologic treatments for youth and to emphasize preventative strategies including regular physical activity. Resistance training (RT) has been suggested as an effective non-pharmacological treatment for the prevention and management of high BP in adults [3,4], yet little is known about the effects of RT on BP in children and adolescents (6–18 years of age) [3].

Research evidence has found that cardiovascular disease has its roots in childhood, with some reports of endothelial damage occurring early in life [5]. The prevalence of diagnosed primary pediatric hypertension is increasing [6,7]. Primary pediatric hypertension is the cardiovascular condition whereby systolic or diastolic BP values are > 95th percentile for boys and girls up to 12 years of age and > 130/80 mmHg for youth older than 13 years of age [6]. Primary pediatric hypertension (as early as 7 years of age) has been associated with pathophysiological changes that tracks into later stages [6,8]. Moreover, the prevalence of obesity is increasing among youth and it has been identified as a risk factor for elevated BP [9,10]. Thus, the prevention and management of obesity early in life should be a primary consideration for reducing the prevalence of pediatric hypertension [9]. Of note, data from diverse populations indicate that childhood BP is associated with BP later in life [11]. Therefore, early treatment and management are needed since accelerated weight gain in youth may increase the risk of elevated BP later in life [12]. Juonala et al. reported that overweight or obesity early in life was predictive of many comorbidities and found that youth who were overweight or obese but who became nonobese as adults had a cardiovascular risk profile that was similar to those who were never obese [13]. Therefore, maintenance of normal body weight in children and adolescents may prevent the clustering of hypertension and other cardiovascular disease risk factors in adulthood [11]. Body mass index (BMI) is the most commonly used surrogate measure of adiposity and screening tool for cardio-metabolic risk [5].

Along with weight maintenance, physical activity can improve BP levels in adults independently of pharmacological treatment [14]. A clinical report demonstrated a decrease in BP values of −5/8 mmHg in hypertensive adults following aerobic training [15]. Traditionally, research and clinical efforts have focused on aerobic training as a means of BP management. Recently, RT has gained attention as an important modulator of BP. Regular participation in RT has been found to reduce BP by −4 mmHg and −5 mmHg in hypertensive adults who performed dynamic and isometric RT, respectively [15].

In addition to increasing muscular strength, muscular power, and local muscular endurance, RT in youth has shown to produce many health benefits including improvements in cardiovascular fitness, body composition, bone mineral density, blood lipid profiles, insulin sensitivity, injury resistance, and mental health [16–24]. By definition, resistance training is a specialized method of conditioning that involves the use of different modes of training with a wide range of resistive loads including body weight exercises and free weights (barbells and dumbbells) [16]. Although the potential health benefits of RT in youth have been widely studied, there is limited understanding about the effects of RT on BP in children and adolescents. Several systematic reviews and meta-analyses have examined the positive effects of RT on BP values in adults. However, no previous systematic review has quantitatively examined the association between RT on BP and BMI in youth. Given this research gap, a systematic review was conducted to examine the literature regarding the effects of youth RT on systolic and diastolic BP. In addition, a meta-analysis of selected studies was conducted to quantitatively evaluate the effects of RT on systolic and diastolic BP, and BMI, in children and adolescents. Given the potential health-related benefits of RT in adults, we hypothesized that RT would also produce beneficial effects on BP and BMI values in youth.

2. Materials and Methods

We followed the recommendations described in the Cochrane Handbook for Systematic Reviews of Interventions version 5.1.0 [25]. Also, the PRISMA statement was used to guide the reporting this Systematic Review (SR) [26] and the protocol for this study was registered in the PROSPERO data base (CRD42020187686).

2.1. Data Sources and Searches

Four electronic databases were searched: PubMed, SPORTDiscus, Web of Science Core Collection and EMBASE to February 2020. No restrictions were set to either publication period or language. The search strategy contained keywords, MeSH terms and Boolean connectors such as AND and OR as follows: [(hypertension OR blood pressure) AND (children OR preadolescents OR youth) AND ("resistance training" OR "weight training" OR "strength training")]. Additionally, included studies and SR on similar topics were reviewed the reference list to find other Randomized controlled trials (RCTS that met the selection criteria.

2.2. Eligibility and Study Selection

After examining the search results, two blinded authors independently assessed the eligibility of all studies retrieved from the databases based on eligibility criteria. Studies were included if they met the following criteria according to patient/problem, intervention, comparison/control or comparator, outcome and study design (PICOS) methodology [25,26]: (i) participants were youth (6–18 years); (ii) the type of study was RCT, (iii) at least one group had to perform RT and (iv) developing RCTs were excluded from this Systematic Review.

2.3. Data Extraction and Quality Assessment

Subject characteristics (i.e., first author's last name; year of publication, age, sex, BMI and training status) and exercise dose were systematically and independently reviewed by two authors (Table 1). For missing data, the correspondence author was contacted by email, requesting information of interest.

2.4. Risk of Bias of Individual Studies

Two review authors worked independently to assessed risk of bias by using domains described in the Cochrane Handbook for Systematic Reviews of Interventions, version 5.1.0 [25]. This set of domains is based on evidence of associations between potential overestimation of effect and the level of risk of bias of the article that may be due to aspects of sequence generation, allocation concealment, blinding, incomplete outcome data, selective reporting. Each criterion was rated as low, high, or unclear risk of bias.

2.5. Data Synthesis and Satistical Analysis

Information on the outcomes of interest was stored in a database. The main results for this study were SBP, DBP and BMI. For continuous outcomes, the group size, the mean values and the standard deviation (SDs) was recorded for each group compared in the included studies. Pooled effects were calculated using an inverse of variance model, and the data were pooled to generate a mean difference (MD) in millimeters of mercury (mmHg) and kilograms on meter squared (kg/m^2) with corresponding 95% confidence intervals (95% CIs). All the studies for each outcome reported data in the same units, so it was possible to pool all studies regardless of whether they reported change data or final data. Significance was set at $p < 0.05$. Statistical heterogeneity was evaluated using the I^2 statistic and classified according to the Cochrane Handbook [25]: negligible heterogeneity, 0% to 40%; moderate heterogeneity, 30% to 60%; substantial heterogeneity, 50% to 90%; and considerable heterogeneity, 75% to 100%. A random-effects model was used. All analyses were performed by one reviewer using Review Manager Version 5.4 and checked against the extracted data by one author.

3. Results

3.1. Literature Search and Article Selection

Initial database searches yielded a total of 1269 articles and the remaining 21 RCTs were found in other sources. After performing screening by title and abstract, and then removing duplicates, a total of 405 research papers were discarded, thus obtaining a total of 32 RCTs for full-text review. Subsequently, 8 RCTs were included in the qualitative synthesis [27–34]. Finally, one author did not respond with missing data, therefore, that study was excluded from the quantitative synthesis. In total 7 studies were included in the meta-analysis [28–34] (Figure 1).

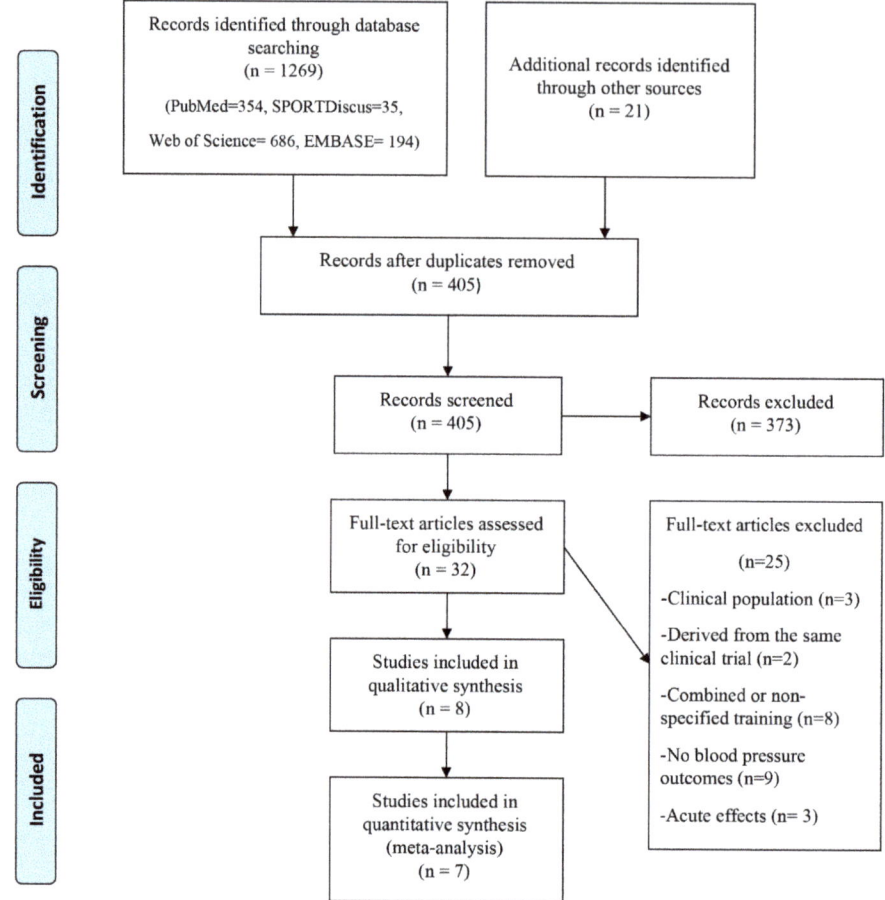

Figure 1. Preferred Reporting Items for Systematic Reviews and Meta-analysis (PRISMA) flow-chart of the study selection.

3.2. Study Characteristics

Eight studies were included in the qualitative analysis, with a total of 8 intervention groups and 571 normotensive or pre-hypertensive youth (intervention group, n = 278; control group, n = 293). The mean of age was 13.28 (2.49) years. Of these, two studies were conducted only with normal weight subjects [27,34], one did not specific it [30], and five realized with obese subjects [28,29,31–33]. The mean of body mass index was 17.26 (35.7) kg/m^2. In addition, in only two of the studies the subjects followed nutritional guidelines [28,31]. One study included only male subjects [29], and another reported the inclusion of exclusively females [27]. The remaining six studies included both sexes. Since blood pressure was not the primary outcome in most studies, there was a great heterogeneity in the measurement procedures. Two studies used a standard sphygmomanometer with cuffs [31,34], two others used an automatic model [28,30] where one was semi-automatic [27] and the other studies did not specify measurement device [29,32,33]. Moreover, significant heterogeneity in the protocols was found ranging from 6 [31] to 40 [30] weeks of RT (Table 1).

Table 1. Resistance Training Studies with Blood Pressure outcome measures.

Source	Population	Intervention Description	BP Assessment Method	Frequency (D/WK)	Intensity	Volume (Sets × REPS)	Study Length (WKS)
Farinatti et al., 2016 [27]	Enrolled: N = 44 Completers: N = 44 44 F; Age: 13–17 Resistance group: N = 24. Obese Control group: N = 20. Non-obese Enrolled N = 81; Completers N = 66 41 M; 40 F; Age: 12–18	RT = chest and leg press, low row, leg extension, upper back, leg and arm curls, leg abduction/adduction, triceps ext.	Semi-automatic sphyngomanometer	3	1–2 Wks: 50–70% 10 RM 3–6 Wks: 60–80% 10 RM 7–12 Wks: 70–85% 10 RM	1 × 15 2 × 8–12 3 × 6–10	12
Horner et al., 2015 [28]	Resistance group: N = 27; 14 M 13 F; Age: 14.6 (1.9) Control group: 24 N = 24; 12 M 12 F; Age: 14.9 (1.8) Enrolled N = 26; Completers N = 26 26 M; Age = 14–18 Obese	RT = Body exercises	automated sphygmomanometer	3	Not report	2 × 12	12
Kelly et al., 2015 [29]	Resistance group: N = 13; Age: 15.4 (0.9) Control group: N = 13; Age: 15.6 (0.96) Enrolled N = 83; Completers N = 83 Age = 8–10	RT = day 1 consisted of compound lower body exercises and isolated upper body exercises and day 2 included com- pound upper body exercises and isolated lower body exercises.	Not report	2	1–4 Wks: light to moderate intensity 5–10 Wks: mod to high intensity 11–16 Wks: mod to high intensity	1 × 10–15 2–3 × 13–15 3–4 × 8–12	16
Larsen et al., 2018 [30]	Resistance group: N = 83 Control group: N = 115	CST = Plyometric and dynamic strength exercises using upper and lower body.	automated sphygmomanometer	3	Not report	30-s all-out exercise periods with 45-s rest periods with 6–10 stations	40

Table 1. Cont.

Source	Population	Intervention Description	BP Assessment Method	Frequency (D/WK)	Intensity	Volume (Sets × REPS)	Study Length (WKS)
Lau et al., 2004 [31]	Enrolled N = 36; Completers N = 36 24 M; 12 F; Age = 10–17 Obese. Resistance group: N = 21 Control group: N = 16 Enrolled N = 23; Completers N = 23 11 M; 12 F; Age = 12–14 Obese.	RT = Lat pull-down, shoulder press, leg press, leg extension, leg curl, heel raise, biceps curl, triceps extension, push-up.	standard mercury sphygmomanometer	3	75–85% RM	1 × 5	6
Naylor et al., 2008 [32]	Resistance group: N = 13; 7 M; 6 F Age: 12.2 (0.4) Control group: N = 10; 4 M; 6 F; Age: 13.6 (0.4) Enrolled N = 304; Completers N = 229 91 M; 213 F; Age = 14–18 Obese	RT = weight-stack machines.	Not report	3	75–90% RM	2 × 8	8
Sigal et al., 2014 [33]	Resistance group: N = 78; 23 M; 55 F; Age: 15.9 (1.5) Control group: N = 76; 24 M; 52 F; Age: 15.6 (1.3) Enrolled N = 38; Completers N = 38 25 M; 13 F; Age = 11–13 Non-obese.	RT = weight machines	Not report	4	65–85% RM	2 × 15	24
Yu et al., 2016 [34]	Resistance group: N = 19; Age: 12.3 (0.42) Control group: N = 19; Age: 12.1 (0.3)	RT = Elbow extension, elbow flexion, trunk extension, trunk flexion, shoulder press, knee extension, knee flexion, push-up, squats, incline dip and hip abd	standard sphygmomanometer	2	12 RM	3 × 12	10

Abbreviations: N, simple size; Female (F), 290; Male (M), 218; RT, resistance training; CST, Circuit Strength Training; D, days; WK, week; WKS, Weeks; REPS, repetitions; RM, maximum repetitions

3.3. Risk of Bias Individual Studies

Three articles clearly report the method of random assignment to the groups [30,33,34]. Only two RCTs describe the allocation concealment [29,33]. In particular, three included studies reported blinding of outcome assessor, the remaining five were judged with unclear risk of bias [32–34]. Additionally, the 8 included RCTs do not describe blinding of study staff and study participants and were judged at high risk of bias for that domain [27–31]. Additional data from the individual analysis of risk of bias is presented in Figure 2.

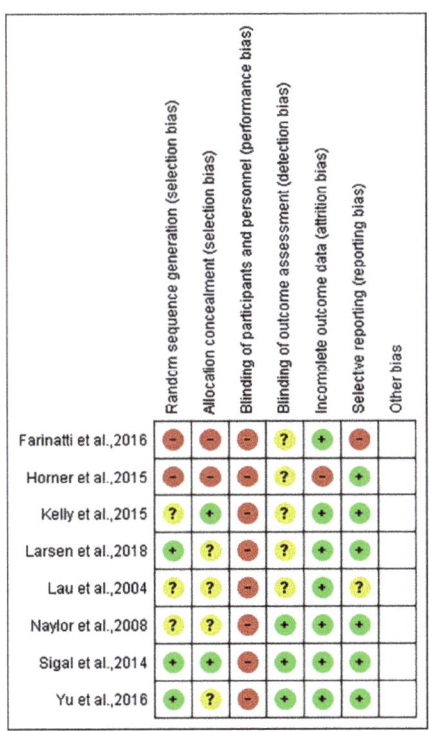

Figure 2. Summary of the risk of bias for the trials included in this meta-analysis. Green indicates low risk of bias, yellow indicated unclear, and red indicates high risk of bias.

3.4. Principle Findings

The results of the meta-analysis showed that no statistically significant reductions were found on the SBP [MD: −1.09 mm Hg (95% CI: −3.24, 1.07), P = 0.32; I^2 = 67%] and the DBP [MD: −0.93 mm Hg (95% CI: −2.05, 0.19), P = 0.10; I^2 = 37%] when comparing the RT groups to the control groups (P = 0.32; P = 0.10, respectively). However, compared to the control group, RT reduced BMI statistically significantly [MD: −0.43 kg/m² (95% CI: −0.82, −0.03), P = 0.03; I^2 = 5%]. Forest plots are presented in Figures 3–5.

Study or Subgroup	Resistance training Mean	SD	Total	Control Mean	SD	Total	Weight	Mean Difference IV, Random, 95% CI
Horner et al.,2015	3.29	13.6	23	1.13	11.9	16	5.8%	2.16 [-5.90, 10.22]
Kelly et al.,2015	-3.8	11.2	13	-5.1	8.3	13	6.4%	1.30 [-6.28, 8.88]
Larsen et al.,2018	2.3	11.6	83	1.1	9.7	115	19.0%	1.20 [-1.86, 4.26]
Lau et al.,2004	-6.4	10.4	21	-0.4	11.6	16	6.9%	-6.00 [-13.22, 1.22]
Naylor et al.,2008	-4	3	13	0	2	10	24.1%	-4.00 [-6.05, -1.95]
Sigal et al.,2014	-4	1	78	-4	1	76	30.5%	0.00 [-0.32, 0.32]
Yu et al.,2016	-3	11	19	-1	11	19	7.3%	-2.00 [-8.99, 4.99]
Total (95% CI)			**250**			**265**	**100.0%**	**-1.09 [-3.24, 1.07]**

Heterogeneity: Tau² = 3.94; Chi² = 18.28, df = 6 (P = 0.006); I² = 67%
Test for overall effect: Z = 0.99 (P = 0.32)

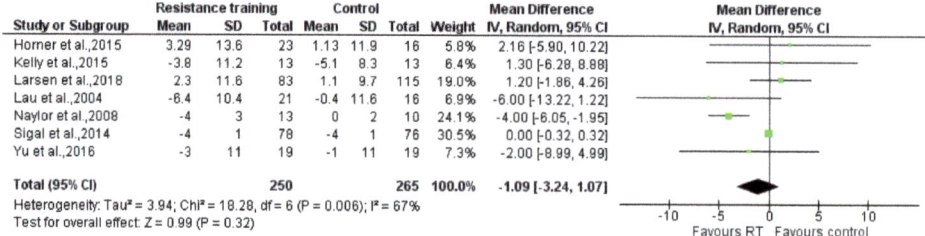

Figure 3. The effect of Resistance Training on systolic blood pressure (mmHg). Total: total number of subjects; CI: confidence interval.

Study or Subgroup	Resistance training Mean	SD	Total	Control Mean	SD	Total	Weight	Mean Difference IV, Random, 95% CI
Horner et al.,2015	0.56	1.61	23	0.08	6.4	16	9.6%	0.48 [-2.72, 3.68]
Kelly et al.,2015	1	9.2	13	0.8	8.55	13	2.5%	0.20 [-6.63, 7.03]
Larsen et al.,2018	-3	6.5	83	0.2	7.9	115	18.4%	-3.20 [-5.21, -1.19]
Lau et al.,2004	-4.2	9.7	21	-1.4	8.9	16	3.2%	-2.80 [-8.82, 3.22]
Naylor et al.,2008	2	3	13	1	2	10	18.0%	1.00 [-1.05, 3.05]
Sigal et al.,2014	-2	1	78	-1	1	76	43.9%	-1.00 [-1.32, -0.68]
Yu et al.,2016	-1	8	19	0	8	19	4.4%	-1.00 [-6.09, 4.09]
Total (95% CI)			**250**			**265**	**100.0%**	**-0.93 [-2.05, 0.19]**

Heterogeneity: Tau² = 0.72; Chi² = 9.54, df = 6 (P = 0.15); I² = 37%
Test for overall effect: Z = 1.63 (P = 0.10)

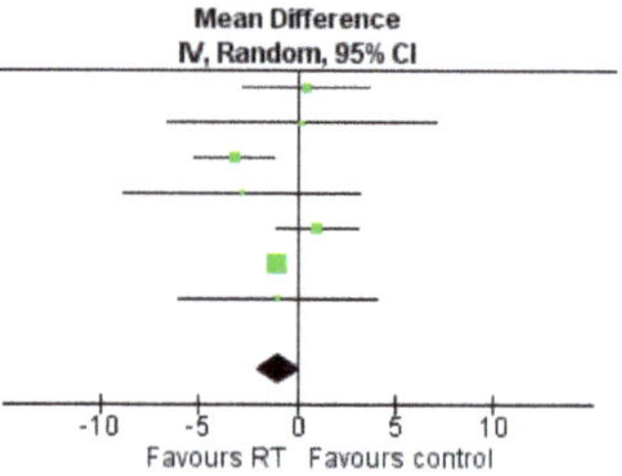

Figure 4. The effect of Resistance Training on diastolic blood pressure (mmHg). Total: total number of subjects; CI: confidence interval.

Study or Subgroup	Resistance training Mean	SD	Total	Control Mean	SD	Total	Weight	Mean Difference IV, Random, 95% CI
Kelly et al.,2015	1.3	6.7	13	-3.6	7.5	13	0.5%	4.90 [-0.57, 10.37]
Lau et al.,2004	-0.1	4.7	21	-0.1	5.4	16	1.4%	0.00 [-3.32, 3.32]
Naylor et al.,2008	-0.6	2	13	-0.2	2.6	10	4.0%	-0.40 [-2.34, 1.54]
Sigal et al.,2014	-0.5	0.6	78	0	0.6	76	87.8%	-0.50 [-0.69, -0.31]
Yu et al.,2016	0.2	2.5	19	0.2	2.3	19	6.3%	0.00 [-1.53, 1.53]
Total (95% CI)			**144**			**134**	**100.0%**	**-0.43 [-0.82, -0.03]**

Heterogeneity: Tau² = 0.04; Chi² = 4.23, df = 4 (P = 0.38); I² = 5%
Test for overall effect: Z = 2.13 (P = 0.03)

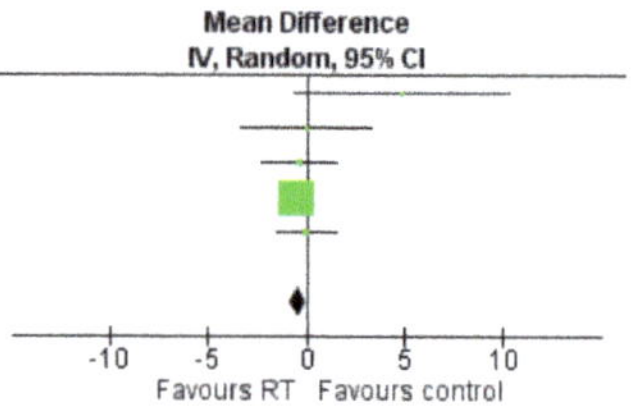

Figure 5. The effect of Resistance Training on body mass index (kg/m^2). Total: total number of subjects; CI: confidence interval.

4. Discussion

The aim of this systematic review and meta-analysis was to quantify the effect of RT on the values of SBP, DBP and BMI in youth. To the best of our knowledge, this is the first systematic review with a subsequent meta-analysis that investigates the effects of RT on BP values in children and adolescents. While other studies have investigated the role of physical activity on cardiometabolic health in youth [35,36], no previous reports have examined the influence of RT in this population. As shown in previous research [3,37], RT has been found to offer observable health-related benefits in adults. Thus, we hypothesized that RT would have positive effects on BP and BMI in youth.

Our main findings are that RT resulted in non significant reductions in SBP (−1.09 mmHg; P = 0.32) and DBP (−0.93 mmHg; P = 0.10) and statistically significant reductions in BMI (−0.43 kg/m^2; P = 0.03) in youth. Although the research reports in this review failed to show statistical significance in terms of the ability of RT to lower systolic and diastolic BP, several factors need to be considered. These factors include the design of the RT protocols (i.e., training intensity, volume, frequency and duration) as well as the health status (all were normotensive) and the training status of the participants. Conflicting findings from several studies are likely due to differences in outcomes measures, study designs and study populations. Regarding the RCTs examined in our review, researchers used different RT protocols. While three studies performed RT with bodyweight exercises [28–30], one used sandbags and dumbbells [34], the others used weight machines [27,31–33]. Notable, there was wide variation in the prescription of RT variables including intensity, volume, frequency or duration. For instance, some protocols proposed two weekly sessions of high RT (12 RM) [34] while others trained 4 days per week with a moderate to high intensity (8 RM) [33]. Further, two studies added nutritional guidelines along with the RT protocol [28,31]. Interpretation and comparison of results would be more accurate with similar RT protocols and with subgroup analysis (i.e., obese and normal body weight; hypertensive and normotensive). There were also differences in the configuration of the control groups among studies that could have impacted the outcomes. For example, two studies did not advise participants about extra physical activity at school or in community based programs [29,33]. In one study that included adolescents who were obese, the control group consisted of adolescents who were not obese [27]. This aforementioned report showed moderate and substantial heterogeneity values in DBP and SBP, respectively (37% and 67%). The heterogeneous values found in this study could help explain why no statistically significant changes were found in SBP and DBP values following RT [27].

RT is an evidence-based preventative exercise intervention strategy that can promote health and well-being through the life course [37,38]. The benefits of progressive RT on muscular strength, muscular power, and local muscular endurance of children and adolescents is well described in several meta-analysis [39–41]. Moreover, RT has shown to produce many health-related benefits including improvements in cardiovascular fitness, body composition, bone mineral density, blood lipid profiles, insulin sensitivity, injury resistance and mental health improvements [16,18–24,42]. Longitudinal studies have confirmed the inverse relationship between low levels of strength early in life and risk of cardiovascular disease later in life [38,43–45]. Therefore, it seems plausible that RT could lower BP concurrent with improvements in other health markers. Some studies have speculated that the reduction in BP following RT in youth might be due to an increase in skeletal muscle mass which, in turn, may lead to a myocardial relaxation [32], diastolic filling peak velocity at the mitral septal annulus [32], an improvement in autonomic modulation [27] and/or an enhanced endothelial function [34]. In obese children, functional and structural cardiac abnormalities (i.e., increased left ventricle and left atrium dimensions, diastolic and systolic left ventricle, and right ventricle dysfunction) have been described in comparison to normo-weight children [46,47]. In this sense, BP mechanisms might be different. Further studies are needed in order to clarify the hypothetical link between RT and BP improvements in youth.

Our findings show a statistically significant improvement in BMI ($P = 0.03$) after an RT intervention. It has been established that exercise interventions can alter body composition (e.g., increase fat free mass) while BMI can remain the same or in some cases increase due to the increase in muscle mass [48]. Indeed, some studies demonstrated no change of BMI following RT despite the remarkable benefits on other health parameters such as endothelial function [49,50]. Therefore, BMI values may underestimate the effectiveness of RT interventions with respect to cardiovascular disease risk [51].

This study has several limitations that should be acknowledged; (1) the lack of systematic quantification of the RT intensity, volume or exercise selection; (2) BP was not a primary outcome in many of the studies included in the analysis; (3) heterogeneity in the outcome measurement procedures; (4) most of the RCTs analyzed did not adequately perform or report random sequence generation, allocation concealment and blinding of outcome assessment and; (5) moderate and substantial values of heterogeneity on SBP and DBP were found.

Although limited research has examined the effects of RT on BP in youth, our results suggest that RT does not have an adverse effect on the BP of children and adolescents and may be beneficial in lowering BP and improving BMI in this young population. Unfortunately, our findings do not allow for a recommendation on a specific dose of RT for effectively managing BP in youth. Nevertheless, a technique-driven and progressive RT program including multijoint exercises that involve the large muscle groups should be considered in the design of youth physical activity programs [16]. Further research is needed to effectively examine the "dose response" (e.g., intensity, volume, frequency) of youth RT interventions while exploring novel modes of RT like low intensity isometric handgrip exercise [52,53].

5. Conclusions

The present shows that there is limited data to determine the effects of RT on BP values in youth, while significant improvements in BMI have been demonstrated. Although the studies show a tendency towards reducing systolic and diastolic BP, the heterogeneity of the RT intensity, volume, frequency or duration make the interpretation of results difficult. Mechanisms by which RT may induce favorable adaptations in BP in youth are speculative. More high-quality studies are needed to clarify the association between RT and BP in youth with and without clinical conditions.

Author Contributions: Conceptualization, C.M.G., I.C.-M.; methodology, C.M.G., A.F.L.-B.; software, A.F.L.-B.; validation, C.M.G., I.C.-M.; formal analysis, A.F.L.-B; investigation, C.M.G., I.C.-M., T.R.R., A.D.F.; resources, C.M.G.; data curation, C.M.G., I.C.-M., T.R.R., A.D.F.; writing-original draft preparation, C.M.G., I.C.-M., A.F.L.-B.; writing-review T.R.R., A.D.F. and editing, C.M.G., A.F.L.-B. I.C.-M., T.R.R., A.D.F.; visualization, C.M.G.; supervision, I.C.-M., T.R.R., A.D.F. All authors have read and agreed to the published version of the manuscript.

Funding: This research received no external funding.

Conflicts of Interest: The authors declare no conflict of interest.

References

1. Hajjar, I.; Kotchen, T.A. Trends in Prevalence, Awareness, in the United States, 1988–2000. *J. Am. Med. Assoc.* **2003**, *290*, 199–206. [CrossRef] [PubMed]
2. Lande, M.B.; Kupferman, J.C. Pediatric hypertension: The Year in Review. *Clin. Pediatr. (Phila)* **2014**, *39*, 57–60. [CrossRef] [PubMed]
3. Cornelissen, V.; Smart, N.A. Exercise Training for Blood Pressure: A Systematic Review and Meta-analysis. *J. Am. Heart Assoc.* **2013**. [CrossRef] [PubMed]
4. Chulvi, I.; Sanchis, J.; Tortosa, J.; Cortell, J.M. Exercise for hypertension. *Fit. Med.* **2016**. [CrossRef]
5. Barlow, S.E. Expert committee recommendations regarding the prevention, assessment, and treatment of child and adolescent overweight and obesity: Summary report. *Pediatrics* **2007**, *120* (Suppl. 4). [CrossRef] [PubMed]
6. Taylor-Zapata, P.; Baker-Smith, C.M.; Burckart, G.; Daniels, S.R.; Flynn, J.T.; Giacoia, G.; Green, D.; Kelly, A.S.; Khurana, M.; Li, J.S.; et al. Research gaps in primary pediatric hypertension. *Pediatrics* **2019**, *143*. [CrossRef] [PubMed]
7. Weaver, D.J. Pediatric hypertension: Review of updated guidelines. *Pediatr. Rev.* **2019**, *40*, 354–358. [CrossRef]
8. Raitakari, O.; Juonala, M.; Nnemaa, T.R.; Kerblom, H.; Viikari, J. Cardiovascular risk factors in childhood as predictors of carotid artery intima-media thickness in adulthood. *Atheroscler. Suppl.* **2003**, *4*, 264. [CrossRef]
9. McMurray, R.G.; Ondrak, K.S. Cardiometabolic Risk Factors in Children: The Importance of Physical Activity. *Am. J. Lifestyle Med.* **2013**, *7*, 292–303. [CrossRef]
10. Falkner, B.; Daniels, S.R. Summary of the fourth report on the diagnosis, evaluation, and treatment of high blood pressure in children and adolescents. *Pediatrics* **2004**, *44*, 387–388. [CrossRef]
11. Chen, X.; Wang, Y.; Chen, X.; Wang, Y. Tracking of Blood Pressure from Childhood to Adulthood A Systematic Review and Meta—Regression Analysis. *Circulation* **2008**, 3171–3180. [CrossRef]
12. Law, C.M.; Shiell, A.W.; Newsome, C.A.; Syddall, H.E.; Shinebourne, E.A.; Fayers, P.M.; Martyn, C.N.; De Swiet, M. Fetal, infant, and childhood growth and adult blood pressure: A longitudinal study from birth to 22 years of age. *Circulation* **2002**, *105*, 1088–1092. [CrossRef] [PubMed]
13. Juonala, M.; Magnussen, C.G.; Berenson, G.S.; Venn, A.; Burns, T.L.; Sabin, M.A.; Srinivasan, S.R.; Daniels, S.R.; Davis, P.H.; Chen, W.; et al. Childhood adiposity, adult adiposity, and cardiovascular risk factors. *N. Engl. J. Med.* **2011**, *365*, 1876–1885. [CrossRef]
14. Williams, B.; Mancia, G.; Spiering, W.; Rosei, E.A.; Azizi, M.; Burnier, M.; Clement, D.; Coca, A.; De Simone, G.; Dominiczak, A.; et al. 2018 practice guidelines for the management of arterial hypertension of the European society of cardiology and the European society of hypertension ESC/ESH task force for the management of arterial hypertension. *J. Hypertens.* **2018**, *36*, 2284–2309. [CrossRef] [PubMed]
15. Arnett, D.K.; Blumenthal, R.S.; Albert, M.A.; Buroker, A.B.; Goldberger, Z.D.; Hahn, E.J.; Himmelfarb, C.D.; Khera, A.; Lloyd-Jones, D.; McEvoy, J.W.; et al. 2019 ACC/AHA Guideline on the Primary Prevention of Cardiovascular Disease: A Report of the American College of Cardiology/American Heart Association Task Force on Clinical Practice Guidelines. *Circulation* **2019**, *140*, e596–e646. [CrossRef] [PubMed]

16. Stricker, P.R.; Faigenbaum, A.D.; McCambridge, T.M. Resistance training for children and adolescents. *Pediatrics* **2020**, *145*. [CrossRef]
17. Faigenbaum, A.D.; Lloyd, R.S.; Myer, G.D. Youth resistance training: Past practices, new perspectives, and future directions. *Pediatr. Exerc. Sci.* **2013**, *25*, 591–604. [CrossRef]
18. Myer, G.; Faigenbaum, A.; Chu, D.; Falkel, J.; Ford, K.; Best, T.; Hewett, T. Integrative Training for Children and Adolescents: Techniques and Practices for Reducing Sports-Related Injuries and Enhancing Athletic Performance. *Phys. Sportsmed.* **2011**, *39*, 74–84. [CrossRef]
19. Lloyd, R.S.; Faigenbaum, A.D.; Stone, M.H.; Oliver, J.L.; Jeffreys, I.; Moody, J.A.; Brewer, C.; Pierce, K.C.; McCambridge, T.M.; Howard, R.; et al. Position statement on youth resistance training: The 2014 International Consensus. *Br. J. Sports Med.* **2014**, *48*, 498–505. [CrossRef]
20. Hind, K.; Burrows, M. Weight-bearing exercise and bone mineral accrual in children and adolescents: A review of controlled trials. *Bone* **2007**, *40*, 14–27. [CrossRef]
21. Bernardoni, B.; Thein-Nissenbaum, J.; Fast, J.; Day, M.; Li, Q.; Wang, S.; Scerpella, T. A school-based resistance intervention improves skeletal growth in adolescent females. *Osteoporos. Int.* **2014**, *25*, 1025–1032. [CrossRef]
22. Ishikawa, S.; Kim, Y.; Kang, M.; Morgan, D.W. Effects of weight-bearing exercise on bone health in girls: A meta-analysis. *Sport. Med.* **2013**, *43*, 875–892. [CrossRef] [PubMed]
23. Lauersen, J.B.; Andersen, T.E.; Andersen, L.B. Strength training as superior, dose-dependent and safe prevention of acute and overuse sports injuries: A systematic review, qualitative analysis and meta-analysis. *Br. J. Sports Med.* **2018**, *52*, 1557–1563. [CrossRef]
24. Collins, H.; Booth, J.N.; Duncan, A.; Fawkner, S.; Niven, A. The Effect of Resistance Training Interventions on 'The Self' in Youth: A Systematic Review and Meta-analysis. *Sport. Med. Open* **2019**, *5*. [CrossRef] [PubMed]
25. Higgins, J.P.T.; Thomas, J.; Chandler, J.; Cumpston, M.; Li, T.; Page, M.J. *Cochrane Handbook for Systematic Reviews of Interventions*; John Wiley & Sons: Hoboken, NJ, USA, 2019.
26. Liberati, A.; Altman, D.G.; Tetzlaff, J.; Mulrow, C.; Gøtzsche, P.C.; Ioannidis, J.P.A.; Clarke, M.; Devereaux, P.J.; Kleijnen, J.; Moher, D. The PRISMA statement for reporting systematic reviews and meta-analyses of studies that evaluate health care interventions: Explanation and elaboration. *J. Clin. Epidemiol.* **2009**, *62*, e1–e34. [CrossRef]
27. Farinatti, P.; Neto, M.; Dias, I.; Cunha, F.A.; Bouskela, E.; Kraemer-Aguiar, L.G. Short-Term Resistance Training Attenuates Cardiac Autonomic Dysfunction in Obese Adolescents. *Pediatr. Exerc. Sci.* **2016**, *28*, 374–380. [CrossRef]
28. Horner, K.; Barinas-Mitchell, E.; DeGroff, C.; Kuk, J.L.; Drant, S.; Lee, S. Effect of Aerobic versus Resistance Exercise on Pulse Wave Velocity, Intima Media Thickness and Left Ventricular Mass in Obese Adolescents. *Pediatr. Exerc. Sci.* **2015**, *27*, 494–502. [CrossRef] [PubMed]
29. Kelly, L.A.; Loza, A.; Lin, X.; Schroeder, E.T.; Hughes, A.; Kirk, A.; Knowles, A.-M. The effect of a home-based strength training program on type 2 diabetes risk in obese Latino boys. *J. Pediatr. Endocrinol. Metab.* **2015**, *28*, 315–322. [CrossRef] [PubMed]
30. Larsen, M.N.; Nielsen, C.M.; Madsen, M.; Manniche, V.; Hansen, L.; Bangsbo, J.; Krustrup, P.; Hansen, P.R. Cardiovascular adaptations after 10 months of intense school-based physical training for 8- to 10-year-old children. *Scand. J. Med. Sci. Sports* **2018**, *28*, 33–41. [CrossRef]
31. Lau, P.W.C.; Yu, C.W.; Lee, A.; Sung, R.Y.T. The physiological and psychological effects of resistance training on Chinese obese adolescents. *J. Exerc. Sci. Fit.* **2004**, *2*, 115–120.
32. Naylor, L.H.; Watts, K.; Sharpe, J.A.; Jones, T.W.; Davis, E.A.N.N.; Thompson, A.; George, K.; Ramsay, J.M.; Driscoll, G.O.; Green, D.J. Resistance Training and Diastolic Myocardial Tissue Velocities in Obese Children. *Med. Sci. Sport. Exerc.* **2008**, 2027–2032. [CrossRef]
33. Sigal, R.J.; Alberga, A.S.; Goldfield, G.S.; Prud'homme, D.; Hadjiyannakis, S.; Gougeon, R.; Phillips, P.; Tulloch, H.; Malcolm, J.; Doucette, S.; et al. Effects of aerobic training, resistance training, or both on percentage body fat and cardiometabolic risk markers in obese adolescents: The healthy eating aerobic and resistance training in youth randomized clinical trial. *JAMA Pediatr.* **2014**, *168*, 1006–1014. [CrossRef] [PubMed]
34. Yu, C.C.-W.; McManus, A.M.; So, H.-K.; Chook, P.; Au, C.-T.; Li, A.M.; Kam, J.T.-C.; So, R.C.-H.; Lam, C.W.-K.; Chan, I.H.-S.; et al. Effects of resistance training on cardiovascular health in non-obese active adolescents. *World J. Clin. Pediatr.* **2016**, *5*, 293–300. [CrossRef] [PubMed]
35. Martínez-Vizcaíno, V.; Pozuelo-Carrascosa, D.P.; García-Prieto, J.C.; Cavero-Redondo, I.; Solera-Martínez, M.; Garrido-Miguel, M.; Díez-Fernández, A.; Ruiz-Hermosa, A.; Sánchez-López, M. Effectiveness of a school-based physical activity intervention on adiposity, fitness and blood pressure: MOVI-KIDS study. *Br. J. Sports Med.* **2020**, *54*, 279–285. [CrossRef]

36. Pozuelo-Carrascosa, D.P.; Cavero-Redondo, I.; Herraiz-Adillo, A.; Diez-Fernandez, A.; Sanchez-Lopez, M.; Martinez-Vizcaino, V. School-based exercise programs and cardiometabolic risk factors: A meta-analysis. *Pediatrics* **2018**, *142*. [CrossRef] [PubMed]
37. Westcott, W.L. Resistance training is medicine: Effects of strength training on health. *Curr. Sports Med. Rep.* **2012**, *11*, 209–216. [CrossRef] [PubMed]
38. García-Hermoso, A.; Ramírez-Campillo, R.; Izquierdo, M. Is Muscular Fitness Associated with Future Health Benefits in Children and Adolescents? A Systematic Review and Meta-Analysis of Longitudinal Studies. *Sport. Med.* **2019**, *49*, 1079–1094. [CrossRef]
39. Behringer, M.; Vom Heede, A.; Yue, Z.; Mester, J. Effects of resistance training in children and adolescents: A meta-analysis. *Pediatrics* **2010**, *126*. [CrossRef]
40. Lesinski, M.; Prieske, O.; Granacher, U. Effects and dose-response relationships of resistance training on physical performance in youth athletes: A systematic review and meta-analysis. *Br. J. Sports Med.* **2016**, *50*, 781–795. [CrossRef]
41. Harries, S.K.; Lubans, D.R.; Callister, R. Resistance training to improve power and sports performance in adolescent athletes: A systematic review and meta-analysis. *J. Sci. Med. Sport* **2012**, *15*, 532–540. [CrossRef]
42. Faigenbaum, A.D.; Kraemer-Aguiar, L.G.; Blimkie, C.J.R.; Jeffreys, I.; Micheli, L.J.; Nitka, M.; Rowland, T.W. Youth Resistance Training: Updated Position Statement Paper From the National Strength and Conditioning Association. *J. Strength Cond. Res.* **2009**, *23*, 60–79. [CrossRef]
43. Ortega, F.B.; Ruiz, J.R.; Castillo, M.J.; Sjöström, M. Physical fitness in childhood and adolescence: A powerful marker of health. *Int. J. Obes.* **2008**, *32*, 1–11. [CrossRef] [PubMed]
44. Grontved, A.; Ried-Larsen, M.; Moller, N.C.; Kristensen, P.L.; Froberg, K.; Brage, S.; Andersen, L.B. Muscle strength in youth and cardiovascular risk in young adulthood (the European Youth Heart Study). *Br. J. Sports Med.* **2015**, *49*, 90–94. [CrossRef] [PubMed]
45. Cohen, D.D.; Gómez-Arbeláez, D.; Camacho, P.A.; Pinzon, S.; Hormiga, C.; Trejos-Suarez, J.; Duperly, J.; Lopez-Jaramillo, P. Low muscle strength is associated with metabolic risk factors in Colombian children: The ACFIES study. *PLoS ONE* **2014**, *9*, e93150. [CrossRef]
46. Alkholy, U.M.; Ahmed, I.A.; Karam, N.A.; Ali, Y.F.; Yosry, A. Assessment of left ventricular mass index could predict metabolic syndrome in obese children. *J. Saudi Hear. Assoc.* **2016**, *28*, 159–166. [CrossRef] [PubMed]
47. Korkmaz, O.; Gursu, H.A.; Karagun, B.S. Comparison of echocardiographic findings with laboratory parameters in obese children. *Cardiol. Young* **2016**, *26*, 1060–1065. [CrossRef]
48. Watts, K.; Jones, T.W.; Davis, E.A.; Green, D. Exercise training in obese children and adolescents: Current concepts. *Sport. Med.* **2005**, *35*, 375–392. [CrossRef]
49. Ferguson, M.A.; Gutin, B.; Owens, S.; Barbeau, P.; Tracy, R.P.; Litaker, M. Effects of physical training and its cessation on the hemostatic system of obese children. *Am. J. Clin. Nutr.* **1999**, *69*, 1130–1134. [CrossRef]
50. Watts, K.; Beye, P.; Siafarikas, A.; O'Driscoll, G.; Jones, T.W.; Davis, E.A.; Green, D.J. Effects of exercise training on vascular function in obese children. *J. Pediatr.* **2004**, *144*, 620–625. [CrossRef]
51. Cote, A.T.; Harris, K.C.; Panagiotopoulos, C.; Sandor, G.G.S.; Devlin, A.M. Childhood Obesity and Cardiovascular Dysfunction. *J. Am. Coll. Cardiol.* **2013**, *62*. [CrossRef]
52. Loaiza-Betancur, A.F.; Pérez Bedoya, E.; Montoya Dávila, J.; Chulvi-Medrano, I. Effect of Isometric Resistance Training on Blood Pressure Values in a Group of Normotensive Participants: A Systematic Review and Meta-analysis. *Sports Health* **2020**, *12*, 256–262. [CrossRef] [PubMed]
53. Loaiza-Betancur, A.F.; Chulvi-Medrano, I. Is Low-Intensity Isometric Handgrip Exercise an Efficient Alternative in Lifestyle Blood Pressure Management? A Systematic Review. *Sports Health* **2020**, *12*, 470–477. [CrossRef] [PubMed]

Publisher's Note: MDPI stays neutral with regard to jurisdictional claims in published maps and institutional affiliations.

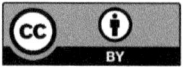

© 2020 by the authors. Licensee MDPI, Basel, Switzerland. This article is an open access article distributed under the terms and conditions of the Creative Commons Attribution (CC BY) license (http://creativecommons.org/licenses/by/4.0/).

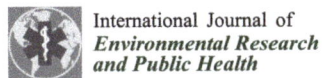 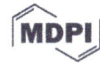

Article

Difficulties of Online Physical Education Classes in Middle and High School and an Efficient Operation Plan to Address Them

Hyun-Chul Jeong [1] and Wi-Young So [2],*

[1] Department of Physical Education, Jeonbuk National University High School, Jeonju-si, Jeollabuk-do 54896, Korea; 01086445918@hanmail.net
[2] Sports and Health Care Major, College of Humanities and Arts, Korea National University of Transportation, Chungju-si 27469, Korea
* Correspondence: wowso@ut.ac.kr

Received: 4 August 2020; Accepted: 2 October 2020; Published: 5 October 2020

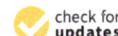

Abstract: This study examined the difficulties of running online physical education classes in the context of coronavirus disease 2019 (COVID-19) and used the findings to develop an efficient operation plan to address these difficulties. Six middle and high school physical education teachers participated; three were experts in online physical education and active in the Korea Council School Physical Education Promotion, and three were recommended teachers making efforts to improve the online classes offered by the Korea Ministry of Education. A qualitative case study method employing phenomenological procedures to collect and analyze the data was used. The difficulties of operating middle and high school online physical education classes for the first time included (1) the monotony of the classes within their limited environmental conditions and limited educational content that did not adequately convey the value of physical education, (2) trial-and-error methods applied nationwide, resulting from a lack of expertise in operating online physical education classes, and (3) very limited evaluation guidelines proposed by the Korea Ministry of Education, which made systematic evaluation with online methods impossible. To address the identified problems and facilitate the efficient operation of online physical education classes, changes in strategic learning methods are needed to understand online physical education characteristics and thereby better communicate the value of physical education. It is also necessary to cultivate teaching expertise through sharing online physical education classes, where collaboration among physical education teachers is central. In addition, evaluation processes should be less formal to encourage active student participation.

Keywords: coronavirus disease-19 pandemic; online evaluation; online physical education class; teaching expertise in physical education; value of physical education

1. Introduction

The entire world is currently facing a catastrophic situation resulting from the coronavirus disease 2019 (COVID-19) pandemic, which has affected the daily lives of people worldwide. Since the World Health Organization declared a pandemic on 11 March 2020, avoiding face-to-face activities and engaging in social distancing have become a part of everyday life. The pandemic has also induced changes in many countries' educational environments as they began instituting online classes, including South Korea (hereinafter Korea), whose schools failed to begin the regular school year in March, for the first time in history. Despite this unprecedented situation, Korea is actively responding to social changes by offering a diverse school curriculum through online classes and developing new approaches to education. The changes required by the crisis may present an opportunity to adapt to the education needs of the incipient Fourth Industrial Revolution. In many studies preceding COVID-19, the possibility of online classes has been examined as a part of future education, in that online classes can provide highly efficient and diverse elective classes to self-directed students [1–6].

Physical education centers on physical activity and is clearly distinct from general knowledge-based subjects. Therefore, online physical education classes require special preparation and operation to communicate and practice the values of physical education well. Currently, as in-person school attendance and online classes are occurring in tandem around the world, there is a need to examine whether online physical education classes are being held and conveying the values of physical education appropriately. Prior studies on the efficiency and potential of online physical education classes, however, are limited [7–9]. One such study focused on physical education textbooks published by the University of North Carolina at Greensboro and suggested employing direct and indirect experiential activities in addition to physical activities [8]. It further proposed a teaching and learning strategy for the management of interaction and motivation, learner-centered classes, and the application of a blended learning strategy in middle school physical education classes [9]. However, most existing studies have only examined the efficiency of college classes, within limited areas; to the best of our knowledge, no studies have investigated the difficulties or efficient operation plans of middle and high school online physical education classes. Thus, there is a need to identify the existing practices of and best directions for future online physical education classes, both during and after the pandemic. This study identifies the difficulties of middle and high school online physical education classes and suggests ways to efficiently manage future online physical education classes. The results may serve as basic material to help revitalize online physical education classes in the future.

2. Materials and Methods

The study employed a qualitative case study method using phenomenological procedures to collect and analyze the data [10]. "Turning to the nature of lived experience" of research participants' online physical education classes, the study explored the experience of conducting these classes, discussed and reflected on their efficient operation and difficulties experienced therein, and examined the data by "writing and rewriting".

2.1. Participants

To find a generalized representation of middle (14–16 years old) and high (17–19 years old) school online physical education classes in Korea, the researcher selected six participants for this study, who were recommended by the Korea Ministry of Education and the Council for School Physical Education Promotion, which pursues the revitalization of physical education in Korea. Three participants were middle and high school physical education teachers who were experts in online physical education; the other three had worked to improve the three types of online classes offered by the Korea Ministry of Education. All participants provided informed consent to participate in the study, which was approved by the Korea Jeonbuk National University High School. Table 1 shows the characteristics of the research participants.

Table 1. Participant characteristics.

Online Physical Education Class Type	School Classes	Role	Gender	Participant	Research Participant Characteristics
Interactive PE Class	"N" Middle School (6 classes)	Teacher	Male	A	As a physical education teacher at "S" Middle School in the 7th year of his educational career, he runs a "Physical Enhancement Program", an interactive PE class of about 20 students, utilizing Zoom. He is a training instructor for online PE content for physical education teachers nationwide and has a good understanding of the pros and cons of interactive PE classes.
	"I" High School (9 Classes)	Teacher	Female	a	As a physical education teacher for "I" High School in the 20th year of her educational career, she runs a "home training and yoga program" using Microsoft Teams, for a class of 15. While operating interactive teacher/student physical education classes, she tries to motivate student participation by using various video content and constantly strives for immediate feedback and interaction with students by asking questions via video.
Content-oriented physical education class	"J" Middle School (32 classes)	Teacher	Female	B	As a physical education teacher for "J" Middle School in the 11th year of her educational career, she runs a content-oriented physical education class using PPT and Open Broadcaster Software (OBS Studio) programs for a class of 30. She switched to a content-oriented physical education class after initially running an interactive PE class, in which many students found it difficult to participate.
	"J" High School (24 classes)	Teacher	Male	b	As a physical education teacher at "J" High School in the 15th year of his educational career, he runs a content-oriented physical education class using YouTube and videos he has produced for a class of 30. He runs a class that combines theory and practice using physical education textbooks. He also works as a lecturer for the J-region Physical Education Research Association.
Assignment-oriented physical education class	"H" Middle School (23 classes)	Teacher	Male	C	As a physical education teacher at "H" High School in the 23rd year of his educational career, he runs an assignment-oriented physical education class using basic lecture-type content for a class of over 30. In addition to physical activity assignments, he offers online group learning assignments to students and provides feedback during class. Currently, he works as a lecturer in the operation of assignment-oriented physical education classes nationwide.
	"G" High School (30 classes)	Teacher	Female	c	As a physical education teacher at "G" High School in the 4th year of her educational career, she runs an assignment-oriented physical education class for 30 students. The class is interactive and includes feedback from the teacher and focuses on "National Health Gymnastics" and "Creative Gymnastics" developed and practiced by students. The class uses Google Classroom and is equipped with assignment videos and explanations.

PE, physical education.

2.2. Data Collection

The collected data included material directly produced by the research participants and online videos of their physical education classes. In-depth individual and group interviews were conducted to examine experiences emerging in the participants' journals. We examined the participants' personal diaries and their online physical education class operations. Five in-depth individual participant interviews lasting 50–70 min were conducted between March and June 2020. The interviews began with participants describing individual operation plans and were centered on the operation of these cases. Five group interviews lasting 60–90 min were also conducted from April to June 2020, focused on difficulties that were encountered and overcome in the online physical education classes. The group interviews were comprised of open discussions among the research participants, which allowed collaborative and interpretive reflection within a seminar format.

2.3. Data Analysis and Research Authenticity

An inductive category analysis was employed, focusing on open coding, axial coding, and core coding [11]. The researcher worked to understand the overall flow and true meaning of the material through repeated reading. The meanings were classified and grouped by subject and analyzed through technical, reflective, and interpretive writing; then, the relationships between the essential elements of the results were identified to determine the overall structure. Finally, an iterative process of reinterpretation, modification, and integration was applied to ensure that the generated categories reflected the purpose of the study.

To enhance the validity of the study and test the consistency of the findings, a triangulation technique cross-verified data through an in-depth description from various angles using the collected data and the researcher's notes. The derived results were reviewed by the participants to ensure that their meanings were accurately expressed. The quality of the study was ensured through continuous feedback from two qualitative research experts (Professor "S" of "J" University and Professor "L" of "S" University), who reviewed the entire study process.

3. Results

3.1. Difficulties in Running Online Middle and High School Physical Education Classes

3.1.1. Conveying the Value of Physical Education

Difficulties in conveying the value of sports in online physical education classes remained in the modified technical practice. This value included maintaining health through physical activities, cultivating community consciousness through physical activities with friends, and developing sports etiquette through sports participation. Students engaged in online physical education classes often cannot secure enough space to effectively take part in physical activity and also have limited access to supplies and equipment needed to follow online physical education classes. Thus, the participants running the online physical education classes used supplies that were readily available at home, which necessarily reduced the physical education units that could be taught. This led to a shift in focus from competition, which is a major part of in-school physical education, to health and physical activity challenges in online instruction.

> Teacher "A": *In online physical education classes, students had to participate alone and use the supplies at home, so it was inevitable that classes were limited. However, it was easy for me to give feedback because I run a real-time interactive class and students practice it immediately in line with my fitness program.*

> Teacher "C": *Real-time interactive classes can be effectively used in a small class, but it seems inefficient in a class of about 30 students. Thus, I used lecture-type content to provide explanations and demonstrations, present assignments, and give feedback.*

> Teacher "b": *I run a content-oriented class, but I had doubts about whether the values of physical education that we wanted to deliver were being conveyed well, given the limited environment and the fact that students had to practice alone.*

> Teacher "c": *I agree. I had actually planned a class in the competition area, but I could only do classes in the health area. I was worried that the students would feel too complacent about physical education through such classes.*

> Teacher "a": *I had no choice but to run really monotonous classes like juggling and "challenging" stay-at-home challenges that could be done in students' own houses.*

(From the first group interview).

In contrast to the general knowledge focus of core subject courses, physical education focuses on physical activity, an emotional domain. All participants had concerns about how to convey physical activities in online physical education classes and how to make the online physical education class a meaningful educational activity. In a study of physical activity limitation, Kim et al. [12] reported that various physical educational activities geared toward health should be included in an online class, as most participants, despite various ages and genders, had health problems.

It is possible that online physical education classes can be made more efficient if students receive feedback through viewing their own or their classmates' actions. This is in contrast to face-to-face physical education classes, where students can immediately receive feedback on their motor skills or their success completing physical activities. In contrast, students cannot modify their own activities by viewing a video of them, so they receive limited feedback. Immediate feedback is needed to motivate students to learn and strengthen their active class attitude. The participants tried to provide feedback across time and space through online media; however, this was difficult, because basic rapport between the teacher and the students and among the students themselves was not able to develop well through the online approach. In addition, the lack of interaction between the teacher and students in online courses made it difficult to convey the value of physical education.

There was an interaction between teachers and students when the teacher provided feedback by checking students' online assignment performance. This interaction became an advantage of interactive physical education classes and assignment-oriented physical education classes. However, this was difficult because basic rapport was not developed through the online approach. In addition, the lack of interaction between the teacher and students in online courses made it difficult to convey the value of physical education.

(From the in-depth interview of Teacher "a").

Like the result of the in-depth interview with Teacher "a," the interaction between the teacher and the student becomes an important factor for the realization of the value of physical education. This experience suggests that attempts to convey the value of physical education should be initiated later in the semester, after rapport has been developed between the teacher and their students and after the technical skills for various sports have been reviewed [13].

3.1.2. Lack of Teacher Experience

Online physical education classes, instituted nearly worldwide during the 2020 pandemic, were a wholly new experience for both teachers and students. The sudden shift to online classes left teachers unprepared and struggling with unfamiliar teaching methods, forcing them to resort to trial-and-error approaches. Inadequate online teaching strategies and low teacher and student readiness for online classes made the transition difficult [14].

I had to think about the content of physical education classes that I could do online with the start of online classes due to COVID-19, and about the content of the class that could be evaluated when students came to school later. The content of online physical education classes were selected based on individual sports that can be done while maintaining social distancing after school starts. However, as the use of various evaluations (individual evaluation, group evaluation, etc.) was limited due to restrictions on class activities by group, I was very worried about what to do. (From the in-depth interview of Teacher "b").

The filming and production of online class materials by the physical education teacher himself took two to three times longer to prepare (e.g., production and editing) than the existing physical education classes. Even if various content (YouTube, Internet materials, etc.) was used, it took a lot of time and effort to search for videos and materials that matched the teaching content of the physical education teacher's class. (From the in-depth interview of Teacher "C").

The participants' principal concerns about running online physical education classes centered on the lack of efficient content and difficulties in using the content. They worried about the students' ability to participate in sufficient physical activities given space restrictions and the online course content they created, and whether the course content was educationally meaningful. The availability of media to capture and edit various physical activity photos and videos was absolutely essential for online course preparation. The participants experienced considerable confusion in their initial attempts at online instruction, although the Ministry of Education and the municipal and provincial education offices provided guidance and training on operating online classes and copyright issues after the switch to online classes.

> *I feel that it is more important than anything else for physical education teachers to develop their ability to efficiently use content in the areas where various aspects of physical activity are expressed and where the content of explanation, demonstration, and feedback is provided. This is an important point that I realized while lecturing in the content utilization training course due to the fact that physical education is unlike the general subjects. I believe that my experience in online physical education classes will definitely be an opportunity.* (From the research journal of Teacher "A").

> *The physical education teachers had to revise their education plans, courses, and evaluations several times in their online physical education classes. It is true that it is very confusing. I am going through a lot of difficulties because it is my first time using the content of online physical education classes and making evaluations.* (From the in-depth interview of Teacher "B").

Physical education teachers who were familiar with online content could easily incorporate it. However, others had difficulties even with simple tasks, such as uploading lectures and linking videos from different sites. Those who developed their own lectures experienced difficulties preparing for online physical education classes, because they lacked the necessary equipment (cameras, microphones, laptops, etc.), had no access to software for editing images and coding video files, and/or lacked experience in using such software. To maximize the efficiency of online physical education classes, both teacher effort and collaboration with online experts were essential [7].

3.1.3. Evaluation

The Ministry of Education presented guidelines for evaluating online classes [15], which specified that teachers were to refrain from conducting evaluations unless they could be done face-to-face and recommended conducting evaluations after the return to in-class instruction to the extent possible. Participants found it difficult to apply evaluations to online physical education classes. It seemed unreasonable to evaluate students on what they had learned in school following a long period of online classes—especially if these were conducted solely through lectures and assignments without the students actually performing and practicing the activities to be evaluated—particularly because the proportion of the evaluation based on physical activity was high, given the nature of the subject of physical education. This differs from general subject evaluations, where written examinations based on online course work can be administered after the return to in-school classes. Although students could submit physical education performance evaluations in the form of videos and written assignments, it would be very time-consuming for large schools to determine whether students had submitted the evaluation materials and then to actually evaluate those materials.

> *In order to evaluate a gymnastics movement, I asked the students to take a picture of themselves doing the gymnastics movement and upload it. However, there were limits in uploading the entire gymnastic movement, and so the evaluation was made in partial movements. In addition, there was too much restriction in providing feedback and evaluation for all images.* (From the in-depth interview of Teacher "c").

> *It has been a while since online physical education classes started, but I don't believe that the performance evaluation proposed by the Ministry of Education is a concrete plan yet. Evaluations must be done in terms of efficiency and expandability of online physical education classes.* (From the in-depth interview of Teacher "B").

Teacher "c", who had been conducting performance evaluations based on assignments, found it difficult to complete the evaluations, because performance assessment was not conducted in real time. In addition, she felt that the diversity and specificity of the evaluation was very poor because they were limited to evaluating individual activities through videos. Each study participant completed evaluations according to the type of online physical education classes they conducted, and all participants described encountering specific difficulties in completing the evaluations.

> Teacher "A": *It is very difficult to check the performance of what students practiced in real-time interactive classes.*
>
> Teacher "a": *The home training and yoga practice scenes were evaluated in real time, but the evaluation took too long.*
>
> Teacher "B": *The performance assignment was checked through simple quizzes and discussions during the content-oriented class, but there were many difficulties in evaluating the actual activities and conducting detailed evaluations.*
>
> Teacher "b": *I believe that the evaluation is essential for online physical education classes. For self-directed learning, the evaluation parts associated with the assignment should be presented in various forms.*
>
> Teacher "C": *Many teachers spend too much time giving feedback and evaluations in assignment-oriented classes. Systematic supplementation is needed online.*
>
> Teacher "c": *Since there is a very limited amount of information that can be recorded in the Student Record in the existing evaluation, a new evaluation method that can evaluate and record the learning process should be introduced.*

(Summary of the discussion on evaluations in the second and third group interviews).

In the second and third group interviews, participants discussed the difficulties of the evaluation and argued that evaluation concepts and practices for online physical education classes should be re-established based on the current evaluation results. They likewise argued that these concepts and practices should include measures that confirm whether students actively participated in the online physical education classes. In addition, physical activity content that can be viewed online needs to be expanded.

3.2. A Plan for the Efficient Operation of Middle and High School Online Physical Education Classes

3.2.1. Content that Conveys the Value of Physical Education

Online physical education classes need to teach the value of physical activity as an important element of health [16]. However, before teaching students the value of physical education, teachers should focus on physical education concepts while preparing students to actively participate in the online class. Online physical education classes should teach students to subjectively develop future physical activity plans and self-directed competencies. Although the internet delivers classes without time and space constraints that nearly everyone can access, such classes are ineffective and inefficient if students do not actively and responsibly participate. In other words, the students' attitude toward self-directed learning is an important factor in the efficient operation of online physical education classes. Therefore, teachers need to develop educational strategies for online classes that help students form a learning attitude. Engaging and motivating students to participate in physical activities can help convey the value of physical education [17].

> Teacher "b": *When conducting training for teachers, the issue was raised that no matter how much effort is made by the teacher to conduct a good class, it will be of no use if the students are not willing to listen. In such a case, the plan needs to be re-examined.*

Teacher "C": Yes, that is correct. If the online physical education class begins and no assignments are given, it would not be possible to check if the student is listening to the online class. Actually, some students do assignments without listening to assignments, which means you can set a group for the class and complete the group work outside of class. Thus, I have tried interactive classes among students to complete a set of assignments as a group.

Teacher "A": That's a good idea. Before discussing the value of physical education, it should be preceded by many educational devices and materials so that students can listen to online classes with an attitude toward self-directed learning.

Teacher "B": Yes, I agree. The value of physical education should be naturally achieved in class, and a good class will be meaningless if the students do not have active learning attitudes.

Teacher "c": Yes, I have tried to make changes in the existing physical education class by making students submit reports and videos based on their activities to make them actively participate in class. (From the fourth group interview).

In the group interviews, participants discussed the buzz learning method as a way to increase student participation in online classes [18]. Changes are essential for developing and applying group assignments that encourage student participation to overcome the disadvantage of online physical education classes [18]. New assignment content needs to be developed in the future that will allow teachers to identify an individual student's learning status, just as the research participants developed different educational strategies to increase the value of the class. Physical activity does not necessarily need to be central in the actual class to establish the value of physical education; Park et al. [19] reported that the establishment of the value of physical education based on various types of materials is necessary in online physical education classes, as various audiovisual aids and activity equipment are provided to support the positive health behavior of university students. There is a need to develop ways to link the emotional areas while expanding the cognitive and defining areas, which can be an advantage of online physical education classes.

Teacher "b" made great efforts to motivate and interest students by using physical education textbooks to explain theoretical aspects and presenting images to help students understand the material. Indirect experience based on direct experience of physical activity and the value of physical education were delivered through intensive classes in cognitive areas using physical education textbooks. (Analyzing the content of Teacher "b's" online physical education class).

I do not think that it is necessary to teach the value of physical education centered on physical activity. Rather, I think that by running this online physical education class, I was able to deliver the value of integrating various topics through theoretical classes in physical education textbooks. I tried to convey the value of physical education by using various video images, arguments, discussions, and reporting that were not well utilized in existing physical education classes. (From the in-depth interview of Teacher "b").

Online physical education classes are clearly different from traditional physical education classes. Participants made changes while running online physical education classes and conveyed the value of physical education in different ways.

3.2.2. Efforts to Cultivate Teacher Expertise

Participants pointed out that one change driven by online physical education classes was the active progress made by physical education teachers through collaboration, which provided training and help to teachers who had difficulty creating content in the early stage of online classes. This collaboration naturally expanded as they produced class videos and shared ideas on assignment methods and structures and class content. This collaboration was driven by the power of collective intelligence within the physical education community and demonstrated a culture of sharing based on the autonomy of the Physical Education Research Society and networks among colleagues [20].

> *Considering that this is my first online class this year, the most distinguishing feature is that there is a place where physical education teachers from a variety of schools share the materials, content, and concerns regarding online physical education classes. Would you say that we were tightly united in a crisis? It seems to have served as an opportunity for physical education teachers to reduce the trial-and-error and to develop better physical education classes.* (From the in-depth interview of Teacher "C").

> *The research participants' videos showed that physical education teachers collaborated on making demonstrations and teaching, thereby producing more professional content by producing a joint video that fit the class subject.* (From the researcher's journal).

The importance of the teacher learning community is reported in many studies on the development of teacher expertise [21–23]. Physical education class videos continue to be produced and teachers continue to cultivate their expertise as they develop and produce these class videos. Research participants continued to develop their expertise by searching for educational materials, including carefully examining materials from The Council School Physical Education Promotion and the Physical Education Research Society, while developing online physical education classes. They further developed their expertise by producing and editing their own videos. The results of their efforts provide a good example of how to effectively prepare for future physical education.

> *I was at a loss when I first started preparing for online physical education classes, but I received a lot of help from the teachers at the Physical Education Research Society. In addition, it really helped me cultivate my expertise while reflecting on my class. It was also very helpful to be able to view the classes of other physical education teachers, which used to be hard to see before.* (From the in-depth interview of Teacher "a").

> *It was great to be able to look at the really valuable materials in The Council School Physical Education Promotion and the National Physical Education Teacher Group's "katokbang". It was good to see many physical education teachers collaborate and build their expertise in "an opportunity that lies in a crisis". That is why I became confident in my class, too.* (From the in-depth interview of Teacher "c").

Physical education teachers who strive to improve their expertise give students faith in the subject. Faith creates interdependence through communication between the teacher and the students and also acts as an "invisible bridge" in physical education classes [24]. Faith between the teacher and students can also be indirectly formed by the teacher's demonstrating instructional content and expertise while running an online class. Efforts are needed to cultivate professional and practical knowledge suitable for online physical education classes through changes in teaching and learning methods, interaction with students, a broad understanding of the area, and expanded knowledge.

3.2.3. Preparation for Improved Evaluations

Online physical education performance is difficult to evaluate. Traditional evaluations are extremely limited, including online and offline integrated evaluations, process-oriented evaluations, and physical activity-oriented evaluations. The research participants adapted their evaluation methods to determine whether the student achievement standards were met and whether advancement to the next class was appropriate.

> *Teacher "A": Teacher evaluation is conducted by looking directly at the student's activities. Peer evaluation is conducted by students looking at one another.*

Teacher "a": Our evaluation method entails showing various videos that fit the topic of the class and talking about the feelings they elicit in real time.

Teacher "B": There is no direct evaluation, and the achievement standards are reviewed by looking at the class and simply writing the overall content in the form of a report.

Teacher "b": A self-assessment is conducted to determine whether the student has participated in class with an attitude toward self-directed learning, and whether the student has completed the assignments, but they are not reflected in the student's score.

Teacher "C": Evaluations cannot be made because it is an assignment-oriented class. Images of the student's physical activity are used to deliver feedback through student self-assessment and teacher evaluation.

Teacher "c": Based on the attached content of assignments carried out by the student, the course is recorded in the physical education section of the student's Study Record.

(Summary of evaluation discussion in the fourth and fifth group interviews).

One characteristic of online education is that students can develop unique thinking through learning activities that meet their needs and cultivate creativity through the process of thinking [25]. Evaluation methods need to be improved to capture the process of verbalizing students' thoughts. It is necessary to conduct evaluations in the form of an inspection to understand the educational value of online physical education classes, much like the way in which the research participants expanded the evaluation to assess diagnosis, formation, and achievement in addition to performance.

The above student faithfully carried out the assignments regarding national health gymnastics during online physical education classes, understood and analyzed teacher and peer evaluation feedback, and faithfully participated in the assignments. (From the examples of Study Records by Teacher "c").

Teacher "A" evaluated interactive lessons in real time, but emphasis was placed on the students who delivered feedback and made corrections according to the feedback. In addition, a peer evaluation method was applied to the class in which feedback was provided by watching videos that in real-time interactive class, meaning other students watch the monitor video between students through informal evaluation. (Analyzing the content of Teacher "A's" online physical education class).

Research participants used informal evaluations to record student participation in the Study Record as a way to induce active participation. This was done while using the performance evaluation content required in physical education classes as a learning strategy. Evaluation of the online classes, which was conducted for the first time in 2020, is not yet concrete, and efficient evaluation methods and content should be examined in future studies.

4. Discussion

This study examined the difficulties teachers experienced in running online physical education classes following the start of online schooling in Korea in the context of COVID-19 and presented an efficient operation plan for future online physical education classes.

The difficulties of operating online middle and high school physical education classes included monotony related to limited environmental conditions and educational content, which ultimately decreased the effectiveness of conveying to students the value of physical education. It is necessary in this light to discuss the value of physical education during online classes. Second, physical education teachers across the country lacked expertise in employing online content and had to resort to trial-and-error methods. To address problems like these, we expect that effective content will develop in various directions due to the COVID-19 outbreak. Third, student evaluations conducted in accordance with the evaluation guidelines proposed by the Korea Ministry of Education were very limited, and a systematic evaluation was not possible because of the online nature of the classes. There is a possibility that a new evaluation method that can be operated effectively in online classes will need to be constructed.

In addition, to develop effective online physical education classes, strategic learning methods that incorporate online physical education characteristics are needed to help teachers communicate the value of physical education. In delivering the values of physical education, which is the goal of physical education in Korea, addressing the psychodynamic domain and affective domain, which are lacking in online classes, will certainly improve the efficiency of online physical education classes. Second, physical education teachers need to prepare for the future methodology of physical education and acquire professional practical knowledge through sharing online physical education content. This collaboration among physical education teachers is central and should incorporate expertise from the Korea Physical Education Research Society. Third, it is necessary for students to make an effort to actively participate in online physical education classes and record the process in their life record books through discussion of evaluation methods and methods suitable for an online physical education class.

In this study, the research participants did not have extensive experience in information and communication technology coming into the pandemic and the advent of online education, but they nevertheless actively participated in online physical education classes and played the role of representatives of Korea, making the active efforts required by the times. Finally, the need is apparent to explore various cases of online physical education, teachers' and students' experiences, and their meaning, to improve the generalizability of the lessons learned.

5. Conclusions

The study findings had several implications. First, it is necessary to study the state of different countries' experiences in online instruction physical education instruction, comparing and analyzing how online physical education classes are conducted worldwide. Accordingly, there is a need to review and systematize approaches to online physical education classes that highlight each country's cultural and educational characteristics and to examine the effectiveness of online physical education classes as a whole. Second, there is a need to explore the potential of online physical education classes linked to face-to-face physical education classes to examine their respective effectiveness and potential possibilities in light of physical education teachers' increased expertise gained through their operation of online physical education classes. Third, future studies should establish a theoretical framework for online physical education classes by examining the educational value of modifying existing pedagogical methods, content, evaluations, and so on to more effectively teach online physical education classes. Fourth, future studies should also examine the efficiency and affordances of different online platforms employed by physical education teachers and evaluate their generalizability across actual school sites, especially as novel tools are developed.

Author Contributions: Study design: H.-C.J. Study conduct: H.-C.J. and W.-Y.S. Data collection: H.-C.J. Data analysis: H.-C.J. Data interpretation: H.-C.J. and W.-Y.S. Drafting the manuscript: H.-C.J. Revising the manuscript content: W.-Y.S. All authors have read and agreed to the published version of the manuscript.

Funding: This research received no external funding.

Conflicts of Interest: The authors declare no conflict of interest.

References

1. Blaine, A.M. Interaction and presence in the virtual classroom: An analysis of the perceptions of students and teachers in online and blended Advanced Placement courses. *Comput. Educ.* **2019**, *132*, 31–43. [CrossRef]
2. Son, C.H.; Kang, S.G.; Ha, S.J. Study on application of online instruction for enhancing rights for learning: Focusing on high schools. *J. Creat. Inf. Cult.* **2016**, *2*, 9–22.

3. Lee, E.J. A study on college students' perception on convenience in online courses. *J. Educ. Inf. Media* **2010**, *16*, 341–362.
4. Lee, N.H.; Jung, H.R. The effects of the flipped learning sensory integration therapy class using online learning platform on learning participation. *Korean Enterainment Ind. Assoc.* **2018**, *12*, 247–256. [CrossRef]
5. Yong, N. On-line classroom visual tracking and quality evaluation by an advanced feature mining technique. *Signal Process. Image Commun.* **2020**, *84*, 115817.
6. Jeong, Y.S. Providing high school students with online instruction for optional curriculum. *Korea Contents Soc.* **2014**, *14*, 500–508. [CrossRef]
7. Lm, H.J.; Kim, S.J. Development and application of e-learning contents to pre-service physical education teacher education. *Korean J. Sport Pedagog.* **2007**, *14*, 21–40.
8. Lyu, M.J. A case study on structure and possibility of online courses in physical education. *J. Res. Curric. Instr.* **2011**, *15*, 353–370.
9. Hong, S.H. A study on teaching and learning plan of physical education in middle school using blended learning strategy linked. *Korean J. Phys. Educ.* **2006**, *45*, 387–402.
10. Van Manen, M. *Researching Liver Experience*; The University of Western Ontario: London, ON, Canada, 1990.
11. Strauss, A.; Corbin, J. *Basics of Qualitative Research: Grounded Theory Procedures and Techniques*, 2nd ed.; Sage: Thousand Oaks, CA, USA, 1998.
12. Kim, S.E.; Lee, Y.S.; Lee, J.Y. Differences in causes of activity limitation by sex and age. *J. Men's Health* **2020**, *16*, e18–e26. [CrossRef]
13. Guan, B. Determination of China's online physical education object. *Procedia Eng.* **2012**, *29*, 3557–3561. [CrossRef]
14. Do, J.W. An investigation of design constraints in the process of converting face-to-face course into online course. *J. Educ. Cult.* **2020**, *26*, 153–173.
15. Korea Ministry of Education. *Guidelines for Attending, Evaluating and Recording Remote Classes to Respond to Corona 19*; Korea Ministry of Education: Sejong, Korea, 2020.
16. Marilyn, M.B.; Jacalyn, L.L.; Joyce, M.H.; Connie, B.C. *Instructional Strategies for Secondary School Physical Education*; McGraw-Hill College: New York, NY, USA, 2006.
17. Ahn, Y.O. Inquiry on justification of the physical education on the view of value theory. *Korean Soc. Elem. Phys. Educ.* **2019**, *25*, 1–18. [CrossRef]
18. Lee, Y.J.; Gwak, B.C. The need of buzz learning in real-time distance education. In Proceedings of the Korean Society of Computer Information Conference, Pusan, Korea, 11 July 2012; Volume 20, pp. 457–458.
19. Park, S.U.; Ahn, H.; So, W.Y. Developing a model of health behavior intentions and actual health behaviors of Korean male university students. *J. Men's Health* **2020**, *16*, e1–e9. [CrossRef]
20. Jeong, H.C.; Kim, D.J. Exploration of culture and meaning of participation in secondary physical education study group. *J. Educ. Cult.* **2018**, *24*, 311–330. [CrossRef]
21. Yoon, K.J.; Lee, G.S.; Lee, C.H. A case study of using an online cafe in a physical education teacher learning community. *Korean J. Sport Pedagog.* **2018**, *25*, 21–40. [CrossRef]
22. Jo, K.H.; Lee, O.S. An investigation of the impacts and factors influencing elementary teachers' participation in a physical education teacher learning community. *Korean J. Phys. Educ.* **2016**, *55*, 251–263.
23. Vangrieken, K.; Meredith, C.; Packer, T.; Kyndt, E. Teacher communities as a context for professional development: A systematic review. *Teach. Teach. Educ.* **2017**, *61*, 47–59. [CrossRef]
24. Jeong, H.C.; Kim, D.J. A self-study on the management experience of learner-centered physical education. *Korean J. Sport Pedagog.* **2020**, *27*, 139–157. [CrossRef]
25. Berge, Z. Characteristics of online teaching in post-secondary, formal education. *Educ. Technol.* **1997**, *37*, 35–47.

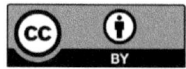

© 2020 by the authors. Licensee MDPI, Basel, Switzerland. This article is an open access article distributed under the terms and conditions of the Creative Commons Attribution (CC BY) license (http://creativecommons.org/licenses/by/4.0/).

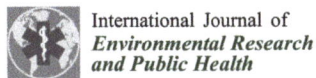

Article

Placing Greater Torque at Shorter or Longer Muscle Lengths? Effects of Cable vs. Barbell Preacher Curl Training on Muscular Strength and Hypertrophy in Young Adults

João Pedro Nunes [1,*], Jeferson L. Jacinto [2], Alex S. Ribeiro [1,2], Jerry L. Mayhew [3], Masatoshi Nakamura [4], Danila M. G. Capel [2], Leidiane R. Santos [2], Leandro Santos [1], Edilson S. Cyrino [1] and Andreo F. Aguiar [2]

1. Metabolism, Nutrition, and Exercise Laboratory, Physical Education and Sport Center, Londrina State University, Londrina 86057-970, PR, Brazil; alex.sribeiro@kroton.com.br (A.S.R.); leandro.santos.sm@gmail.com (L.S.); edilsoncyrino@gmail.com (E.S.C.)
2. Center for Research in Health Sciences, University of Northern Paraná, Londrina 86041-140, PR, Brazil; jeferson1995lucas@gmail.com (J.L.J.); danilamcapel@gmail.com (D.M.G.C.); leydremigio@gmail.com (L.R.S.); afaguiarunesp@gmail.com (A.F.A.)
3. Exercise Science Program, Truman State University, Kirksville, MO 63501, USA; jmayhew@truman.edu
4. Niigata University of Health and Welfare, Niigata 950-3198, Japan; masatoshi-nakamura@nuhw.ac.jp
* Correspondence: jaaonunes@gmail.com

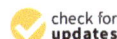

Received: 11 July 2020; Accepted: 10 August 2020; Published: 13 August 2020

Abstract: Muscular strength and hypertrophy following resistance training may be obtained in different degrees depending on the approach performed. This study was designed to compare the responses of the biceps brachii to two preacher curl exercises, one performed on a cable-pulley system (CAB; in which a greater torque was applied during the exercise when elbows were flexed and biceps shortened) and one performed with a barbell (BAR; in which greater torque was applied when the elbows were extended and biceps stretched). Thirty-five young adults (CAB: 13 men, 5 women; BAR: 12 men, 5 women; age = 24 ± 5 years) performed a resistance training program three times per week for 10 weeks, with preacher curl exercises performed in three sets of 8–12 repetitions. Outcomes measured included elbow flexion peak isokinetic torque at angles of 20°, 60°, and 100° (considering 0° as elbow extended), and biceps brachii thickness (B-mode ultrasound). Following the training period, there were significant increases for both groups in elbow flexion peak torque at the 20° (CAB: 30%; BAR = 39%; $p = 0.046$), 60° (CAB: 27%; BAR = 32%; $p = 0.874$), and 100° (CAB: 17%; BAR = 19%; $p = 0.728$), and biceps brachii thickness (CAB: 7%; BAR = 8%; $p = 0.346$). In conclusion, gains in muscular strength were greater for BAR only at longer muscle length, whereas hypertrophy was similar regardless of whether torque emphasis was carried out in the final (CAB) or initial (BAR) degrees of the range of motion of the preacher curl in young adults.

Keywords: variable resistance; muscle architecture; exercise selection; strength training; Scott curl

1. Introduction

Depending on the purpose of the resistance training program, specific adjustments in the training schedule should be made [1]. Whilst the effects of some variables, such as training volume and intensity, have been widely investigated, exercise selection to elicit specific effects on muscle has not [2]. It is worth noting that exercise selection in resistance-training programs is generally based on acute biomechanical studies [2,3]. However, given the gap between acute and chronic responses, long-term investigations are needed to determine the effects of executing different exercises on primary outcomes of strength and hypertrophy.

For muscular strength, responses are directly dependent on the task practiced [4,5]. That is, regardless of the specific training variable manipulated, more significant performance increases tend to be observed when the strength tests are similar to the exercise task and intensity of load employed during training [5–8]. For example, the benefit of traditional linear periodization programs for improving one-repetition maximum strength seems to be because participants train with higher loads during sessions near post-training evaluation [4]. Moreover, strength adaptations seem to be vector and angle specific, such that greater results tend to be observed in the direction and at the specific angle where higher torque was applied during the execution of the exercise [6,8,9]. For muscle hypertrophy, it seems that the muscle portions that show greater acute activation tend to have greater long-term growth compared to other portions [10–12].

In the same way, a recent review with meta-analysis regarding isometric training indicated that training at longer muscle lengths was superior to training at shorter lengths for improving strength throughout a wide range of motion [13]. Furthermore, it was observed that greater strength gains were obtained in the position trained compared with other tested angles [13], following the specificity principle [14,15]. Moreover, training at longer muscle lengths tended to produce greater hypertrophy [13]. This seems to most likely occur by altering joint moment arm, providing greater mechanical tension [13,16], which has been shown to be important for muscle growth [1]. Given that muscle tends to grow where it experiences the highest levels of tension, and more sarcomerogenesis may occur to adapt the muscle to receive high torques when stretched [16,17], greater hypertrophy in training with elongated muscle would be plausible.

It remains unclear whether strength and hypertrophy changes occur in dynamic exercises when the highest torque application is during different positions of the range of motion. That is to say, will larger strength and hypertrophy gains occur when the highest torque is produced in a specific range of motion? Therefore, this study was designed to compare the responses to two preacher curl exercises, in which maximal force was applied in a shortened or an elongated position following 10 weeks of progressive resistance training in young adults. In order to investigate these points, participants were invited to perform the exercises on a cable-pulley system (CAB), in which a greater torque was applied during the exercise when elbows were flexed and biceps shortened, or with a barbell (BAR), in which greater torque was applied when the elbows were extended and biceps elongated (Figure 1). It was hypothesized that the increase in muscular strength would be angle-specific [13,15], and greater hypertrophy would be observed for the BAR group [13].

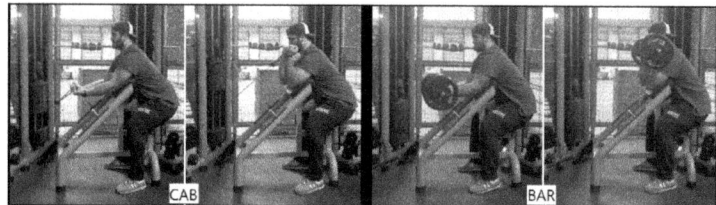

Figure 1. Examples of how cable (CAB) and barbell (BAR) preacher curls were performed.

2. Materials and Methods

2.1. Experimental Design

This study is part of a large research project designed to analyze the effects of whole-body resistance-training protocols in untrained young adults, where participants performed eight exercises, in the following sequence: bench press, leg-press, wide-grip lat-pulldown, leg extension, preacher curl (cable or barbell), leg curl, triceps pushdown, and shoulder lateral raise. The current investigation was executed over a period of 14 weeks, in which weeks 1–2 were used for familiarization with the exercises, week 3 and week 14 were used for pre- and post-training strength and hypertrophy measurements, respectively, and the training program was carried out for 10 weeks (weeks 4–13). During weeks 1–2, participants performed the preacher curl with both the cable and barbell apparatus, alternating between sessions. For the 10-week specific training period, participants were randomly divided into two groups for the CAB or BAR training. Maximum arm flexion strength was assessed on an isokinetic dynamometer, while hypertrophy was analyzed by changes in biceps brachii thickness. Written informed consent was obtained from all participants after a detailed description of study procedures was provided. This investigation was conducted according to the Declaration of Helsinki and was approved by the University Ethics Committee (number: 01993418.9.0000.0108).

2.2. Participants

Recruitment was carried out through social media and home delivery of flyers in the university area. Interested participants completed detailed health history and physical activity questionnaires and were subsequently admitted if they met following inclusion criteria: 18–35 years old, free from cardiac, orthopedic, or musculoskeletal disorders that could impede exercise practice, did not consume drug or supplement ergogenic aids, and not involved in the practice of resistance training over the 6 months before the start of the study. From the 112 volunteers, 74 met the criteria, but only 57 remained after the familiarization period and were evaluated at baseline, and initiated the training sessions. During the training period, participants who obtained six absences from training sessions (resulting in an attendance < 80% of the total number of sessions) were withdrawn from the training program. Thirty-five participants (CAB: 13 men, 5 women; BAR: 12 men, 5 women) ultimately completed the study and were included for final analyses (age = 23.7 ± 5.3 years; body mass = 71.7 ± 12.2 kg; stature = 172.9 ± 8.6 cm; body mass index = 25.0 ± 3.6 kg/m2). This final sample size is considered satisfactory ($n > 16$ per group) to achieve a power of 0.8 and an α of 0.05 for improving muscle morphology with an effect size of 0.50 [18].

2.3. Muscular Strength

Elbow flexion strength was determined from the concentric peak torque (Nm) of the dominant arm, assessed on an isokinetic dynamometer (Biodex Medical Systems Inc., System 3 model, Shirley, MA, USA). Upon arriving at the laboratory, participants were positioned in the sitting position in an 85° hip flexion, according to anatomical position. The axis of the dynamometer lever was aligned with the lateral epicondyle of the humerus. The elbow was supported on a padded shelf with the shoulder flexed at an angle of 60°, similar to the preacher bench. Two straps were secured to keep the torso stabilized. Gravity correction was applied at 0° (parallel to the horizon position), and cushioning was set at moderate, according to the manufacturer's recommendations. During the test, participants were instructed to hold the lever firmly with the hand in a supine position and were admonished to pull it as strongly and quickly as possible. Each participant performed 10 attempts of elbow flexions through a range of motion of 0–120° at an angular velocity of 60°/s, with 3–5 s rest between them. Maximum torques at 20°, 60°, 100° were recorded. Although the test standardized by the equipment was for elbow flexion/extension, participants completed only elbow flexion with maximum force and returned to the starting position (i.e., elbow extensions) by relaxing the limb. Test-retest (separated by 72 h) indicated an intraclass correlation coefficient of 0.95, 0.96, and 0.89, and a standard error of measurement of 3.8 Nm, 3.2 Nm, and 3.1 Nm, for maximum torques at 20°, 60°, and 100°, respectively [19].

2.4. Muscle Thickness

Measures of biceps brachii thickness were obtained using a B-mode ultrasound with a 10.0-MHz linear probe (Esaote, MyLabTM30 model, Florence, Italy) by the same experimenter, blinded to group allocation. Upon arrival at the laboratory on measurement days, participants had to verbally certify that they had been fasting for 8 h and had not performed vigorous exercise for the previous 48 h.

Ultrasound measurements started after participants were lying down in prone position for 10 min. Images were acquired halfway the distance between the acromion process of the scapula and the olecranon process of the ulna. Water-soluble transmission gel was applied over the skin of the muscle being assessed with caution not to depress the muscle tissue. Images were acquired with the probe placed perpendicular to the tissue interface and were recorded at 25 Hz, with a field of view of 60 mm depth. Two experimenters participated in measurement procedures so that one handled the probe, and the other was responsible for freezing the images (once the first considered that image quality was satisfactory). An image as an example of how biceps muscle thickness was measured can be seen in the Supplementary Material. The muscle thickness was defined as the distance between the superficial and deep aponeuroses.

2.5. Preacher Curl Training

The supervised resistance-training program was performed three times per week (Mondays, Wednesdays, and Fridays) in the afternoon period for 10 weeks. This training length has previously been shown to provide adequate time for hypertrophy to occur [18,20,21]. The preacher curl exercises (Ipiranga, Fitness Line, Presidente Prudente, Brazil) were performed in 3 sets of 8–12 repetitions, in the maximum range of motion, in a tempo of 1:2 s (concentric and eccentric phases, respectively). When near to momentary muscular failure (last ~2 repetitions), participants were released to carry out the movement at a capable velocity. The rest between sets was 90–120 s. Training loads were initially selected based on the training logs of the familiarization sessions and were fine-adjusted following a protocol previously described [22,23] so that the participants used a load related to 8–12 RM. Loads were progressively increased each week by ~5%, as recommended [24], according to the number of repetitions performed during training sessions to ensure that the participants kept performing the sets to (or very near to) failure in the established repetition zone [25]. For both groups, participants were instructed to hold the straight handle (or the bar) with hands supinated and shoulder-width apart. Figure 1 illustrates how exercises were performed.

2.6. Statistical Analyses

Normality and homogeneity of variances were checked by the Shapiro–Wilk and Levene's tests, respectively. Non-normal variables (peak torque at 20° and 60°) were analyzed with $\log_{10}$ adjustment. Training effects were examined with analysis of covariance of the raw difference between pre- to postintervention measures, with baseline values as a covariate to eliminate any possible influence of initial score variances on outcomes. Interpretation of data was based on 95% confidence intervals (CI) of the change score (e.g., when the Bonferroni-adjusted 95% CI of the raw delta did not overlap 0, there was a difference between baseline score). The p values of the analysis of covariance for group comparisons were also presented. Additionally, three-way repeated-measures analysis of variance, comparing times (pre vs. post), groups (CAB vs. BAR), and sexes (men vs. women), was performed to determine whether responses to CAB vs. BAR training interacted with sex. A $p < 0.05$ was accepted as statistically significant. Effect size (ES) was calculated as post-training mean minus pretraining mean, divided by pooled pretraining standard deviation [26]. An ES of 0.00–0.19 was considered as trivial, 0.20–0.49 as small, 0.50–0.79 as moderate, and ≥0.80 as large [26]. The data were expressed as mean, standard deviation, and 95% CI. The data were stored and analyzed using JASP software (Jasp Stats, v.1.0. Amsterdam, The Netherlands).

3. Results

No significant time × group × sex interaction was observed for elbow flexion peak torque at 20° ($p = 0.241$; ES of the change: women = 0.78; men = 0.76), at 60° ($p = 0.286$; ES of the change: women = 0.56; men = 0.85), and at 100° ($p = 0.888$; ES of the change: women = 0.42; men = 0.59), nor for biceps muscle thickness ($p = 0.382$; ES of the change: women = 0.35; men = 0.42), indicating that responses to cable or barbell preacher curls were similar between men and women.

For elbow flexion peak torque at 20°, significant increases were observed for both CAB (pre = 30 ± 13 Nm, post = 38 ± 12 Nm; ES = 0.65; +30%) and BAR (pre = 31 ± 14 Nm, post = 42 ± 14 Nm; ES = 0.86; +39%), with greater gains for the BAR group ($p = 0.046$). For elbow flexion peak torque at 60°, significant increases were observed for both CAB (pre = 32 ± 12 Nm, post = 40 ± 12 Nm; ES = 0.73; +27%) and BAR (pre = 30 ± 12 Nm, post = 39 ± 14 Nm; ES = 0.79; +32%), without significant difference between them ($p = 0.874$). For elbow flexion peak torque at 100°, significant increases were observed for both CAB (pre = 31 ± 11 Nm, post = 36 ± 11 Nm; ES = 0.54; +17%) and BAR (pre = 26 ± 9 Nm, post = 32 ± 8 Nm; ES = 0.52; +20%), without significant difference between them ($p = 0.728$). For biceps brachii thickness, significant increases were observed for both CAB (pre = 25 ± 5 mm, post = 27 ± 6 mm; ES = 0.37; +7%) and BAR (pre = 24 ± 4 mm, post = 26 ± 4 mm; ES = 0.35; +8%), without significant difference between them ($p = 0.346$). Individual standardized changes according to groups are displayed in Figure 2.

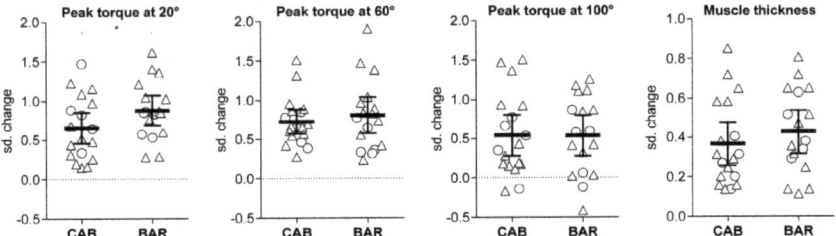

Figure 2. Individual standardized (sd.) changes (post-training minus pretraining value, divided by pooled pretraining standard deviation) for elbow flexion isokinetic peak torque at 20°, 60°, and 100°, and muscle thickness according to groups that performed cable (CAB, $n = 18$) or barbell (BAR, $n = 17$) preacher curl exercises. The horizontal lines represent mean and 95% confidence intervals. Triangles represent men, and circles represent women. * $p < 0.05$ between groups.

4. Discussion

The main finding of the present study was that biceps brachii muscle adaptations following a 10-week training program were almost identical regardless of whether peak torque emphasis was carried out in the final degrees (CAB) or initial degrees (BAR) of the range of motion in young adults. Our hypothesis that greater strength and hypertrophy would occur when peak toque was generated early in the range of motion was not confirmed. A significant advantage, albeit of small magnitude (ES = 0.23), was observed for BAR on improving extended elbow strength (at 20°) compared to CAB, which was the portion of the range of motion in which the BAR condition had the greatest torque during exercise, indicating a specificity of the adaptation. However, to comprehensively confirm that strength gains were indeed angle specific, the CAB group should have had a larger increase in peak torque at 100°, which was not the case.

Given that performing isometric training at longer muscle lengths may improve strength to adjacent angles of the trained one [13,14], it can be supposed that BAR induced greater strength gains at 20°, leading to a significant difference compared to CAB, but also prompted gains to the other tested angles. That is, the gains induced by BAR at the angle where CAB would present an advantage (i.e., at 100°) were sufficient to be similar to those obtained by CAB. On the other hand, since training at shorter muscle lengths may give gains that are more angle specific and may not result in significant gains beyond the trained angle [13,14], this propitiated that there was a significant difference between groups in the angle distant (i.e., 20°) to those the CAB trained with greater torque (i.e., ~100°). These findings are very similar to those presented by Thépaut-Mathieu et al. [14] with isometric training. Young male adults trained isometric elbow flexions at 25°, 80°, or 120° for 5 weeks, 3x/week. Strength gains for the 25° group were higher at 25° and similar at 80° compared to the

80°-group. For the 80°-group, responses were greater at 80° and similar at 120° compared to the 120°-group. Similar responses have also been observed in other joints [13].

After the training period, the CAB and BAR groups increased biceps brachii thickness in a similar magnitude, i.e., regardless of the muscle length with which the greater peak of torque was imposed to biceps in the preacher curl. The hypothesis that greater hypertrophy would be observed for the BAR group was not confirmed. The rationale was based on the greater internal physiological stress which would be produced by the muscle at a longer muscle length compared to shorter muscle lengths, due to the difference in moment arm length between conditions. At longer muscle lengths, there are more interactions between actin and myosin filaments, thus, as a result of the increased mechanical stress placed on the elongated muscle, greater hypertrophy would occur [13,16,27,28], which was not the case herein. However, on the other hand, greater metabolic stress may be obtained when focusing the exercise execution training with short lengths [29]. Thus, the balance between lower and greater torque at the distinct phases of the movement (i.e., lower torque for CAB and greater for BAR at the initial angles; and vice-versa) and between mechanical and metabolic stress—which are factors, among others, important for muscle growth [1]—may explain the similarity of results between CAB and BAR.

Previous findings also on biceps brachii, from Pinto et al. [20], showed similar hypertrophy following preacher curl at full (0–130°) and partial (50–100°) ranges of motion. Conversely, studies on the quadriceps muscle indicated hypertrophic benefits to training at longer muscle lengths [27,30]. After lower-limb training at longer (40–90° of knee flexion; 0° = full knee extension) and shorter (0–50°) muscle lengths, McMahon et al. [30] observed a benefit on vastus lateralis hypertrophy (at the proximal, middle, and distal sites) for the longer-length training condition. However, in another experiment, after training protocols at longer (0–90° of knee flexion) and shorter (0–50°) average muscle lengths, the authors showed an evident advantage for training at longer muscle lengths only at the distal site of the vastus lateralis [27]. Together, these results indicate that a clear benefit for training at long muscle lengths may occur only when training in that length in an isolated manner, and in comparison to shorter isolated ones [13,16,20,27,29,30]; so that the slight difference produced by the present exercise setups was not sufficient to elicit different adaptations.

The present study has some issues to be addressed. Firstly, the training program included other exercises for the elbow flexors, and this, despite having a high relation to practical settings, might have clouded the true magnitude of the effect of preacher curl training [21]. Moreover, this experiment was carried out in untrained young adults and results cannot be generalized to other populations of different ages, or training statuses, given that responses to training are influenced by such factors [1,24]. Finally, muscle thickness was assessed only at the mid-portion of the biceps, and considering that training-induced hypertrophy may be inhomogeneous [1,17,31], the assessment of more muscle sites (e.g., proximal and distal; short and long heads of the biceps separately) might provide greater insights regarding the hypertrophy responses.

5. Conclusions

In conclusion, similar responses to preacher curl training were obtained with CAB and BAR apparatus. The BAR group obtained greater strength gains at 20° of the elbow flexion, while no difference was observed between groups for strength gains at the 60° and 100° positions and the muscle thickness.

The results of this study suggest that coaches and practitioners can choose to perform preacher curl training on a cable-pulley device or with a barbell with the expectation of achieving similar results for strength and hypertrophy. The choice may be based on the availability of equipment or personal preference. If one apparatus is occupied in the weight room, the other can be utilized without diminishing the training effects. Combining both approaches may also be a valid strategy. Moreover, although extrapolations should be done with caution, other similar exercise variations (e.g., lying chest flies on low-pulley cable vs. dumbbells) with which the highest torque is during the final or initial degrees of the movement may induce similar adaptations (to the pectoralis major, for example) as well.

Supplementary Materials: The following are available online at http://www.mdpi.com/1660-4601/17/16/5859/s1, Figure S1: Overview of the measure of the thickness of biceps brachii muscle.

Author Contributions: Conceptualization, J.P.N., J.L.J., A.S.R., J.L.M., M.N., L.S., E.S.C. and A.F.A.; Formal analysis, J.P.N.; Investigation, J.P.N., J.L.J., A.S.R. and A.F.A.; Methodology, J.P.N., J.L.J., A.S.R., E.S.C. and A.F.A.; Project administration, J.P.N., J.L.J. and A.F.A.; Supervision, J.P.N., J.L.J., D.M.G.C., L.R.S. and L.S.; Writing—original draft, J.P.N.; Writing—review & editing, J.P.N., J.L.J., A.S.R., J.L.M., M.N., D.M.G.C., L.R.S., L.S., E.S.C. and A.F.A. All authors have read and agreed to the published version of the manuscript.

Funding: This research received no external funding.

Acknowledgments: The authors would like to express thanks to all the participants for their engagement in this study, the Coordination of Improvement of Higher Education Personnel (CAPES/Brazil) for the scholarship conferred to J.P.N. (master), and the National Council of Technological and Scientific Development (CNPq/Brazil) for the grants conceded to E.S.C. This study was partially supported by the Ministry of Education (MEC/Brazil) and CNPq/Brazil.

Conflicts of Interest: The authors declare no conflict of interest.

References

1. Schoenfeld, B.J. The Mechanisms of Muscle Hypertrophy and Their Application to Resistance Training. *J. Strength Cond. Res.* **2010**, *24*, 2857–2872. [CrossRef] [PubMed]
2. Ribeiro, A.S.; Nunes, J.P.; Schoenfeld, B.J. Selection of Resistance Exercises for Older Individuals: The Forgotten Variable. *Sports Med.* **2020**, *50*, 1051–1057. [CrossRef] [PubMed]
3. Krause Neto, W.; Soares, E.G.; Vieira, T.L.; Aguiar, R.; Chola, T.A.; Sampaio, V.L.; Gama, E. Gluteus maximus activation during common strength and hypertrophy exercises: A systematic review. *J. Sport Sci. Med.* **2020**, *19*, 195–203.
4. Nunes, J.P.; Ribeiro, A.S.; Schoenfeld, B.J.; Cyrino, E.S. Comment on: "Comparison of Periodized and Non-Periodized Resistance Training on Maximal Strength: A Meta-Analysis". *Sports Med.* **2018**, *48*, 491–494. [CrossRef]
5. Schoenfeld, B.J.; Grgic, J.; Ogborn, D.; Krieger, J.W. Strength and hypertrophy adaptations between low— versus high-load resistance training: A systematic review and meta-analysis. *J. Strength Cond. Res.* **2017**, *31*, 3508–3523. [CrossRef]
6. Buckner, S.L.; Jessee, M.B.; Mattocks, K.T.; Mouser, J.G.; Counts, B.R.; Dankel, S.J.; Loenneke, J.P. Determining Strength: A Case for Multiple Methods of Measurement. *Sports Med.* **2017**, *47*, 193–195. [CrossRef]
7. Brandão, L.; Painelli, V.D.S.; Lasevicius, T.; Silva-Batista, C.; Brendon, H.; Schoenfeld, B.J.; Aihara, A.Y.; Cardoso, F.N.; Peres, B.D.A.; Teixeira, E.L. Varying the Order of Combinations of Single- and Multi-Joint Exercises Differentially Affects Resistance Training Adaptations. *J. Strength Cond. Res.* **2020**, *34*, 1254–1263. [CrossRef]
8. Contreras, B.; Vigotsky, A.D.; Schoenfeld, B.J.; Beardsley, C.; McMaster, D.T.; Reyneke, J.H.; Cronin, J.B. Effects of a Six-Week Hip Thrust vs. Front Squat Resistance Training Program on Performance in Adolescent Males: A randomized controlled trial. *J. Strength Cond. Res.* **2017**, *31*, 999–1008. [CrossRef]
9. Bloomquist, K.; Langberg, H.; Karlsen, S.; Madsgaard, S.; Boesen, M.; Raastad, T. Effect of range of motion in heavy load squatting on muscle and tendon adaptations. *Graefe's Arch. Clin. Exp. Ophthalmol.* **2013**, *113*, 2133–2142. [CrossRef]
10. Nunes, J.P.; Costa, B.D.; Kassiano, W.; Kunevaliki, G.; Castro-E-Souza, P.; Rodacki, A.L.; Fortes, L.S.; Cyrino, E.S. Different Foot Positioning During Calf Training to Induce Portion-Specific Gastrocnemius Muscle Hypertrophy. *J. Strength Cond. Res.* **2020**, *34*, 2347–2351. [CrossRef]
11. Wakahara, T.; Fukutani, A.; Kawakami, Y.; Yanai, T. Nonuniform Muscle Hypertrophy: Its relation to muscle activation in training session. *Med. Sci. Sports Exerc.* **2013**, *45*, 2158–2165. [CrossRef] [PubMed]
12. Hirono, T.; Ikezoe, T.; Taniguchi, M.; Tanaka, H.; Saeki, J.; Yagi, M.; Umehara, J.; Ichihashi, N. Relationship Between Muscle Swelling and Hypertrophy Induced by Resistance Training. *J. Strength Cond. Res.* **2020**. [CrossRef]

13. Oranchuk, D.J.; Storey, A.G.; Nelson, A.R.; Cronin, J.B. Isometric training and long-term adaptations: Effects of muscle length, intensity, and intent: A systematic review. *Scand. J. Med. Sci. Sports* **2019**, *29*, 484–503. [CrossRef]
14. Thépaut-Mathieu, C.; Van Hoecke, J.; Maton, B. Myoelectrical and mechanical changes linked to length specificity during isometric training. *J. Appl. Physiol.* **1988**, *64*, 1500–1505. [CrossRef] [PubMed]
15. Lanza, M.B.; Balshaw, T.G.; Folland, J.P. Is the joint-angle specificity of isometric resistance training real? And if so, does it have a neural basis? *Graefe's Arch. Clin. Exp. Ophthalmol.* **2019**, *119*, 2465–2476. [CrossRef]
16. Noorkoiv, M.; Nosaka, K.; Blazevich, A.J. Neuromuscular Adaptations Associated with Knee Joint Angle-Specific Force Change. *Med. Sci. Sports Exerc.* **2014**, *46*, 1525–1537. [CrossRef]
17. Nunes, J.P.; Schoenfeld, B.J.; Nakamura, M.; Ribeiro, A.S.; Cunha, P.M.; Cyrino, E.S. Does stretch training induce muscle hypertrophy in humans? A review of the literature. *Clin. Physiol. Funct. Imaging* **2020**, *40*, 148–156. [CrossRef] [PubMed]
18. Schoenfeld, B.J.; Ogborn, D.; Krieger, J.W. Dose-response relationship between weekly resistance training volume and increases in muscle mass: A systematic review and meta-analysis. *J. Sports Sci.* **2017**, *35*, 1073–1082. [CrossRef]
19. Hopkins, W.G. Spreadsheets for analysis of validity and reliability. *Sport Sci.* **2015**, *19*, 36–42.
20. Pinto, R.S.; Gomes, N.; Radaelli, R.; Botton, C.E.; E Brown, L.; Bottaro, M. Effect of Range of Motion on Muscle Strength and Thickness. *J. Strength Cond. Res.* **2012**, *26*, 2140–2145. [CrossRef]
21. Mannarino, P.; Matta, T.; Lima, J.; Simão, R.; De Salles, B.F. Single-Joint Exercise Results in Higher Hypertrophy of Elbow Flexors Than Multijoint Exercise. *J. Strength Cond. Res.* **2019**. [CrossRef] [PubMed]
22. Nunes, J.P.; Marcori, A.J.; Tomeleri, C.M.; Nascimento, M.A.; Mayhew, J.L.; Ribeiro, A.S.; Cyrino, E.S. Starting the Resistance-Training Session with Lower-Body Exercises Provides Lower Session Perceived Exertion without Altering the Training Volume in Older Women. *Int. J. Exerc.Sci.* **2019**, *12*, 1187–1197. [PubMed]
23. Ribeiro, A.S.; Avelar, A.; Schoenfeld, B.J.; Fleck, S.J.; De Souza, M.F.; Padilha, C.S.; Cyrino, E.S. Analysis of the training load during a hypertrophy-type resistance training programme in men and women. *Eur. J. Sport Sci.* **2015**, *15*, 256–264. [CrossRef]
24. Kraemer, W.J.; Adams, K.; Cafarelli, E.; A Dudley, G.; Dooly, C.; Feigenbaum, M.S.; Fleck, S.J.; Franklin, B.; Fry, A.C.; Hoffman, J.; et al. American College of Sports Medicine position stand. Progression models in resistance training for healthy adults. *Med. Sci. Sports Exerc.* **2009**, *41*, 687–708.
25. Dankel, S.J.; Jessee, M.B.; Mattocks, K.T.; Mouser, J.G.; Counts, B.R.; Buckner, S.L.; Loenneke, J.P. Training to Fatigue: The Answer for Standardization When Assessing Muscle Hypertrophy? *Sports Med.* **2017**, *47*, 1021–1027. [CrossRef]
26. Cohen, J. A power primer. *Psychol. Bull.* **1992**, *112*, 155–159. [CrossRef]
27. McMahon, G.; Morse, C.I.; Burden, A.M.; Winwood, K.; Onambélé, G.L. Impact of Range of Motion During Ecologically Valid Resistance Training Protocols on Muscle Size, Subcutaneous Fat, and Strength. *J. Strength Cond. Res.* **2014**, *28*, 245–255. [CrossRef]
28. Rassier, D.; MacIntosh, B.R.; Herzog, W. Length dependence of active force production in skeletal muscle. *J. Appl. Physiol.* **1999**, *86*, 1445–1457. [CrossRef]
29. Goto, M.; Maeda, C.; Hirayama, T.; Terada, S.; Nirengi, S.; Kurosawa, Y.; Nagano, A.; Hamaoka, T. Partial Range of Motion Exercise Is Effective for Facilitating Muscle Hypertrophy and Function Through Sustained Intramuscular Hypoxia in Young Trained Men. *J. Strength Cond. Res.* **2019**, *33*, 1286–1294. [CrossRef]
30. McMahon, G.; Morse, C.I.; Burden, A.; Winwood, K.; Onambélé, G.L. Muscular adaptations and insulin-like growth factor-I (IGF-I) responses to resistance training are stretch-mediated. *Muscle Nerve* **2013**, *49*, 108–119. [CrossRef]
31. Antonio, J. Nonuniform Response of Skeletal Muscle to Heavy Resistance Training: Can bodybuilders induce regional muscle hypertrophy? *J. Strength Cond. Res.* **2000**, *14*, 102–113. [CrossRef]

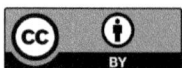

© 2020 by the authors. Licensee MDPI, Basel, Switzerland. This article is an open access article distributed under the terms and conditions of the Creative Commons Attribution (CC BY) license (http://creativecommons.org/licenses/by/4.0/).

MDPI
St. Alban-Anlage 66
4052 Basel
Switzerland
Tel. +41 61 683 77 34
Fax +41 61 302 89 18
www.mdpi.com

International Journal of Environmental Research and Public Health Editorial Office
E-mail: ijerph@mdpi.com
www.mdpi.com/journal/ijerph

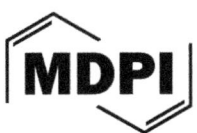

www.ingramcontent.com/pod-product-compliance
Lightning Source LLC
LaVergne TN
LVHW070609100526
838202LV00012B/602